QUANTUM FIT
Be wise be fit

SUDARSHAN

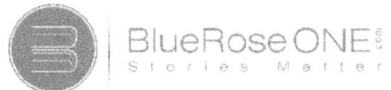

© Sudarshan 2023

All rights reserved

All rights reserved by author. No part of this publication may be reproduced, stored in a retrieval system or transmitted in any form or by any means, electronic, mechanical, photocopying, recording or otherwise, without the prior permission of the author.

Although every precaution has been taken to verify the accuracy of the information contained herein, the author and publisher assume no responsibility for any errors or omissions. No liability is assumed for damages that may result from the use of information contained within.

First Published in May 2023

ISBN: 978-93-5741-516-3

BLUEROSE PUBLISHERS

www.bluerosepublishers.com
info@bluerosepublishers.com
+91 8882 898 898

Cover Design:
Yash

Typographic Design:
Tanya Raj Upadhyay

Distributed by: BlueRose, Amazon, Flipkart

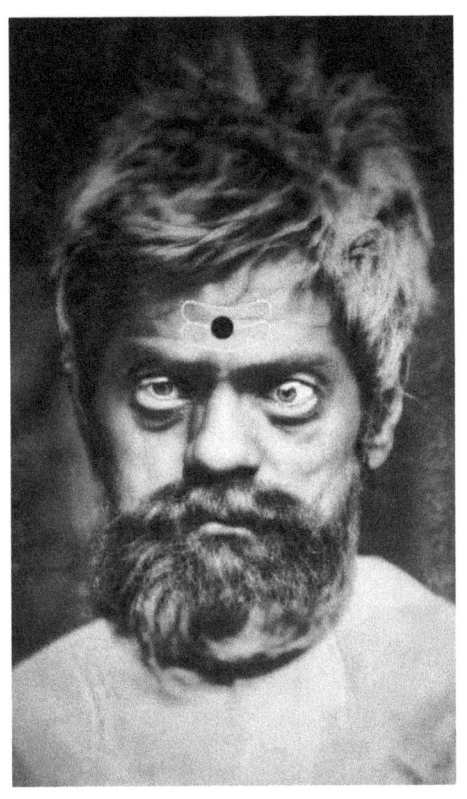

My 1st book is dedicated to the 'SOURCE'
- Sadguru Shankar Maharaj

Table of Contents

Fitness 1
Wise Description of Fitness 4
Aspects of Fitness 15
Wise Aspects of Fitness 18
Type of Workouts commonly known 24
Wisely categorized types of Workouts 27
General Sequence of Workouts 53
Wise sequence of workouts 105
Ideal workout suggestions as per Ayurvedic wisdom considering 'Tridoshas' 120
Wise understanding about the 'Process of Results' 127
Preparation to start your Fitness Routine 143
Pre-requisites of Workout 160
Body Exercise Mechanism 162
Precautions of Restarting after a long gap 165
Understanding Human Body in terms of Waves, Vibrations and Frequencies 169
Electromagnetic Field of Human Body and Mother Earth 172
Golden Ratio and Human Body Design 177
Understand Functioning of Human Body 181
Connect and energize yourself to the nature through basic elements 188

Beyond Imagination	210
The '4S' Formula	222
Break the Ice	236
Benefits of Exercise	238
Body Weight and Confusion	248
Importance of Fitness and Health	275
Strengths and Weaknesses	276
Genetics and Fitness	278
Good Habits – Bad Habits	283
Age and Fitness	290
Oxidative Stress	294
Lifestyle and Fitness	297
Immunity and Exercise	300
Beauty in Simplicity	304
Give sufficient required Time and Keep Patience	306
Consistency, Discipline and Progression	309
Realistic Fitness Goal	313
Unrealistic Fitness Goals	315
Types of Recoveries	317
Importance of Stretches in recovery	323
Lactic Acid and its effect on recovery	325
Matured Perspective towards Health and Fitness	328
Nothing Is Good in Excess – Achieve a great Balance in Everything	333

Fitness

Fitness can be referred to be the ability to perform physical activity and maintain good health. It involves the combination of various physical and mental attributes, such as strength, endurance, flexibility, and balance, that help an individual lead a healthy and active lifestyle.

Fitness can be improved through regular exercise, proper nutrition, and adequate sleep. The most common forms of physical activity that contribute to fitness are cardiovascular exercise, strength training, and flexibility exercises.

Fitness is important for overall health as it helps prevent various diseases, improves mental health, and increases lifespan. It also helps maintain a healthy weight, improves bone density, and reduces the risk of injury.

Achieving and maintaining fitness requires a balanced and consistent approach, combining regular exercise with a healthy Nutrition intake and a healthy lifestyle. This may include eating a well-balanced nutritious food, reducing stress, and avoiding harmful habits such as smoking and excessive alcohol consumption etc.

Fitness goals can vary greatly from person to person, ranging from losing weight to improving athletic performance. It is important to set realistic and achievable goals, and to track progress towards these goals in order to stay motivated. Always start with small and easy to maintain, steps in the beginning.

There are many different types of fitness programs and activities to choose from, so it is important to find a program that is right for you. Whether you prefer individual or group activities, indoor or outdoor activities, or low-impact or high-impact activities, there is something for everyone. A wise and sensible choice considering multiple factors always matters and become beneficial in long run.

Fitness can be improved at any age, and it is never too late to start. With the right combination of exercise, nutrition, and lifestyle choices, anyone can achieve and maintain good fitness, irrespective of Age and gender.

It is important to consult not just with a doctor, but also an experienced fitness coach or expert before starting any new fitness program, especially if you have any pre-existing medical conditions or injuries. A doctor can help you determine the best approach for your specific needs and goals. Similarly, a well experienced fitness coach/ expert will surely help you to find out and decide your temporary needs as well as short term and long-term goals, by a thorough and detailed consultation and also by considering different important factors which have been affecting your health and fitness so far and which could possibly affect your fitness journey in long run.

A knowledgeable and experienced personal trainer can also be a great resource for guidance and support. They can help you design a customized fitness plan, provide tips for injury prevention, and help you stay motivated and on track towards your fitness goals by clearing your basic ideas and by making your routine the simplest to follow yet effective.

Thus, fitness is the most crucial aspect of overall health and wellness. Whether you are just starting out or are a seasoned fitness enthusiast, taking the time to prioritize fitness can lead to a happier, healthier, and more fulfilling life.

So, never underestimate your 'Me Time' i.e., your 'Workout Session' in a day and lose the opportunity to keep yourself Fit. Because Consistency is the key to open the Lock of Abundant Fitness, Health and Wellness in a great divine order.

Wise Description of Fitness

As per the scientific definition, most of the people think that fitness is very specific about the body Weight, Body Fat, Body Shape, Lean muscles, More strength, More stamina and Flexibility. But these are just the superficial observations of the changes happening in the body with a constant effort on exercise, nutrition and rest. These observations are generally taught and preached by most of the fitness professionals to the common people as per their own knowledge and understanding about 'Fitness'. Most of the time fitness is considered about the difference achieved in visibility or the measurable changes happening in the body.

There is much more depth and meaning, beyond these typical and Common observations and parameters about fitness. People should increase the reach of their level of understanding, thoughts and acceptance with a matured and broader approach towards the term 'fitness' in today's time.

Fitness can be explained at physical levels, psychological levels and beyond. We may even consider the external aspects which includes our surroundings, nature and the universe itself. Similarly, we may consider the internal aspects right from the cell levels, all the internal organs, systems and their functions, also we can consider our fitness at emotional levels, mental or psychological levels. We may consider fitness at the spiritual level too.

In short, it's all about the connection. The connection in between our physical body, mind and soul. And our connection with others, that means with other humans, animals, different species, these species may include many types of bacterial bodies which are not visible to human eyes but they are present inside our body as well as in the nature or in our surroundings and different entities carrying different types of energies. So, we deal with all these things in our day today life knowingly or unknowingly. Connection with surroundings, nature and the entire universe and the connection with one's own self has its own significance. Connection with own self and understanding our own self and understanding the purpose of our existence can be called as 'Self Realization'. Self-Realization is Ability to understand our actual role in this huge system in which we exist.

This connection might be very effective, average, or very weak, similar to a mobile phone and the network of the sim card inside it. The same way, this connection might be different depending on different aspects and also on an individual's body, mind, and soul. The important thing is that how effectively and efficiently we connect with our own selves, with our family, friends, our pets, our surroundings, or with nature all depends on our level of consciousness and fitness, on how physically, psychologically, emotionally, and spiritually fit we are to get a better understanding of our own selves and others and to make this connection more effective and efficient. For this effective connectivity, we need to maintain our physical body very well, because it works as a device for this connection. So, we need to take good care of our body at all levels and maintain a great level of fitness always.

As I mentioned above, we can consider our body a medium or a device to connect with our own selves, other things, our surroundings, nature, or the universe. In order to have a better connection with all of it, or to attract the best of the frequencies and vibes, we need to keep this device properly maintained. And for maintenance, we need to do physical exercises that cover all aspects, including strength, stamina, flexibility, and better mind-muscle coordination, i.e., internal connectivity, communication, and coordination between the brain, heart, and physical body. Also detoxifying, by removing debris, i.e., different types of acids, toxins, biproducts, and by removing excess fat (which is surrounding the internal organs, which badly affect their functions and make the systems very slow), as well as by removing the fat on top of the muscles, we need to achieve an ideal BMI (body mass index) to perform and function at its best, and this is just one parameter. We can even consider 'Mental Detox' because 'negative psychology, negative thoughts, or negative vibes' can be considered as toxins, so it's very important to remove negative thoughts from the mind and always have a positive mindset for positive changes. And the one who achieves all the things mentioned above, achieves the ability to connect with the universe, nature, surroundings, and others as well as with one's own self with complete clarity, then this achievement can be wisely called as 'fitness'.

Nothing is permanent in this world, including 'fitness'.

'Fitness' is always about 'timing'; it is just for the 'time being'. It's about our present or current situation or condition. And it may change. If you are able to maintain consistency in your routine and make progress in it, then your levels of fitness could be considered high. If you barely manage to maintain it, then your levels of fitness could be considered moderate. If you are not putting a single effort into maintaining your fitness, then you are at risk of having low levels of fitness, which is where one should never be, especially in the current 'pandemic' situation. And this 'time being' is always related to your current condition, level, situation, phase. Also, upon your surroundings, lifestyle, and every single aspect related to you on an individual level. And this may differ from time to time or from situation to situation. So, we need to maintain it always, with constant efforts and actual work for it on all levels—physical, psychological or mental, emotional, and spiritual—and there is always a scope for betterment on all levels. So, fitness is not a fixed or constant 'state', and it may not remain forever. You need to earn it first and maintain it, then progress in it, and then maintain that progress with constant efforts, dedication, consistency, hard work, and self-discipline. It's like playing a game on your mobile phone and achieving different levels one by one with constant effort, but there is a twist: in 'Fitness, the game never gets over.

As per one's age, gender, physical ability, disabilities/limitations, fitness goals, present fitness levels, body type, genetic structure and psychology or mind set and even we may consider the surroundings or environment levels of fitness and meaning of fitness or fitness Goals may be different on an individual level.

The actual meaning or definition of 'Fitness' could be different for everyone; it depends purely on individual levels. We may consider the following Examples:

For someone who is physically injured and is in recovery phase, fitness might be just getting out of the bed or standing up from a chair without any struggle and pain for that 'time being'.

- o Fit to Walk – For someone, who is a senior citizen, fitness could be just to walk down the market several blocks away from the house to buy vegetables and fruits and return back with two bags full in both hands, without any fatigue, tiredness or pain.

- Fit to Run – For someone who has a very busy work schedule and have to travel a long way to reach to office by local transport, fitness could be just to run and catch the bus or to run and reach to the platform to catch the train in time.

- Fit to Lift Weights – For someone who is a labour, fitness could be to lift heavy bags or parcels and load on a truck without getting too tired and complete his work shift, as a part of his routine work.

- Fit to Stretch – For someone who is a housemaker and is in her late 40s and can easily pick up some object from the floor with a pain free forward bend, this could possibly the idea of 'Fitness' for her.

- Fit to Balance – For someone who is an electrician and can climb a ladder at the first floor and able to repair a device by maintaining proper balance (Mainly because of Improved Core Strength and alertness, mind muscle co-ordination and great muscle endurance) and successfully completes his work without any risk of losing focus and falling down. And this could be the definition of 'Fitness' for him.

- Fit to do office work – For Someone who is an IT Professional and need to sit and do a desk job for 8-12 Hrs a day in his/her shift. And is able to complete this without any fatigue, stress and imbalance of Muscles or particular joint or Muscle pains and aches.
- Fit to do household work – For someone who is a Housemaker and needs to remember many things and perform and complete many tasks with perfection (which requires a lot of energy) and need to work for longer hours with a lot of patience.
- Fit to Fight Bacterial Infection – For someone who is suffering from any chronic disease or any lifestyle disorder or having weak immune system for years.
- Fit to Give Best Performance – For someone who is an athlete and needs to outperform and win the First Place in his sport on the day of competition.
- Fit to Entertain – For someone who is an entertainer, plays a 'Joker' in a circus and need to give an outstanding performance with full energy and able to leave the entire audience present in the theatre with an uncontrollable Laugh along with abdominal pain and tears in their eyes.

And so on.

One could be always better at work, enhance their performance and become 'Fitter' day by day by adding efforts on the maintenance and progression in their exercise routine on daily basis or at least 4 days a week. There is always a scope. So, we need to focus on a 'Fitness' routine.

A good fitness routine always leads to a great performance and outcome at work.

There could be many more stories and examples of 'Fitness' as per the lifestyle, profession, fitness levels and health conditions related to their respective, surroundings and situations.

So, we need to understand that, it all depends from person to person. Everyone is not living the same life, everyone is not of the same 'make', everyone doesn't have the same surroundings, basically everyone is different internally as well as externally, so 'Fitness' is definitely and always will be different for all, considering different factors.

And 'General Fitness' can be considered Gross.

So, this reminds us about one of the famous trending quotes on social media nowadays, i.e. 'We are not Same Bro!'.

We may also consider the following aspects as 'Wise'

Fitness is a state of physical and mental well-being, achieved through proper exercise and nutrition.

A fit body is not just about having a slim figure or toned muscles, but also about overall health and longevity.

Regular exercise helps improve cardiovascular health, strengthen bones and muscles, boost immunity and increase energy levels.

A balanced diet that includes a variety of whole foods, fruits, vegetables, lean protein and healthy fats is essential for optimal fitness.

Staying fit requires dedication and discipline, but the benefits are endless and include reduced stress, improved self-esteem, and a positive outlook on life.

A combination of strength training and cardiovascular exercise, along with proper rest and recovery, is key to achieving and maintaining fitness.

Fitness is not just about appearance, it's also about functionality and being able to perform daily activities with ease.

Staying fit also helps prevent chronic diseases such as diabetes, heart disease, and certain types of cancer.

Fitness is not a one-time achievement, it is a lifelong journey that requires consistent effort to improve on multiple aspect and have a great balance in between

them, also by keeping faith in the process and with a willingness to adapt the changes at different stages, with a great amount of patience.

Whether you prefer high-intensity workouts or low-impact activities, it's important to find an exercise routine that works for you and fits your lifestyle.

A sedentary lifestyle can have a negative impact on your health and increase the risk of chronic diseases, so it's important to incorporate physical activity into your daily routine. But remember the choice of exercises should be wise considering multiple factors so that it should suit your sedentary lifestyle and support you to maintain the exercise routine with ease.

A healthy body requires not only exercise, but also proper hydration, adequate sleep, and stress management techniques.

Fitness is a journey that requires patience, persistence and a positive attitude always.

Remember to listen to your body and make modifications to your workout routine as needed to avoid injury and ensure progress.

Group fitness classes, personal training, and outdoor activities can add variety and motivation to your fitness routine. A right guidance is always important to make your fitness journey successful.

Fitness is not just about reaching a goal; it's about creating a healthy and fulfilling lifestyle. And know that it is a lifelong process, pay attention, give sufficient time, keep patience and trust the process.

Don't be discouraged by setbacks, embrace them as opportunities to learn and grow. Every step matters.

Surround yourself with positive, supportive people who encourage and motivate you on your fitness journey. Positivity always attracts positivity.

Fitness should be enjoyable and empowering, not a source of stress or anxiety. Do not take any kind of mental stress about your progression, consistency or any kind of goal achievements and never compare yourself with anyone else. You are doing this for your own good, so enjoy every moment of the process.

Whether your goal is to lose weight, build muscle or simply maintain a healthy lifestyle, fitness is a journey that requires dedication, hard work and a positive attitude.

Aspects of Fitness

There are several aspects of fitness, which can be broadly categorized into the following categories:

1. **Cardiovascular endurance:** The ability of the heart and lungs to deliver oxygen to the body during prolonged physical activity.

It is also known as **Cardiorespiratory endurance.** It is the level at which your heart, lungs, and muscles sync and work together when you're exercising for an extended period of time. This shows how efficiently your **cardiorespiratory** system functions, and is an indicator of how physically fit and healthy you are. And this higher level can be achieved through Regular Practice.

2. **Muscular strength:** The ability of muscles to generate force. **Muscular strength** is the amount of force a muscle can produce against Maximum Resistance (As per the Maximum Strength of the Performer) in a single effort (In 1 rep Max – ability to lift maximum weight as per one's capacity for just 1 repetition).

Note: 1 Rep Max is the riskiest thing to think of doing and it probably could be 'Fatal' at times. In my opinion no one should try to attempt it without

any fitness expert's advice, guidance, under observation and most important progressive practice with great consistency over years.

This level can be achieved through regular practice, by fulfilment of Daily Required Nutrition and Sufficient Rest Period for Recovery.

3. **Muscular endurance:** The ability of muscles to perform work over an extended period of time without fatigue. It is the ability of a muscle to repeatedly exert force against resistance. Many factors contribute to **muscular endurance**, including genetics. And this ability of the higher level of performance can be improved by Practicing Technically Correct.

4. **Flexibility:** The ability of joints to move through a full range of motion. **Flexibility** is the range of motion in a joint or group of joints or the ability to move joints effectively through a complete range of motion. **Flexibility** training includes stretching exercises to lengthen the muscles

Regular Practice of **'Yoga'** is the best way to improve on Flexibility.

5. **Ideal Body composition:** The ratio of lean mass to fat mass in the body. **Body composition** is the proportion of **fat** and non-**fat** mass in your **body**. A **healthy body composition** is one that includes a lower percentage of **body fat** and a higher percentage

of non-**fat** mass, which includes muscle, bones, and organs. Knowing your **body composition** one can help you assess your health and fitness level.

By Regular Exercise routine, Sensible Nutrition and Required Rest for recovery can lead to 'Ideal Body Composition' over the period of time.

Here are additional aspects those can be considered too:

1. **Balance:** The ability to maintain control of the body's centre of gravity.
2. **Power:** The ability to generate force quickly.
3. **Speed:** The ability to perform a movement in a short amount of time.
4. **Agility:** The ability to change the direction of the body quickly and accurately.
5. **Coordination:** The ability to perform movements smoothly and efficiently.

    It is important to note that fitness is not just about physical attributes, but also includes mental and emotional wellness, as well as healthy habits and behaviours. A well-rounded fitness program should aim to address all aspects of fitness for optimal health and well-being.

    And that means we are supposed to be **'Quantum Fit'**.

Wise Aspects of Fitness

The "wise aspects of fitness" refers to the various elements that contribute to overall physical wellness and health. It encompasses both the physical and mental aspects of fitness, recognizing that they are interdependent and impact each other in meaningful ways.

- ❖ **Physical fitness**: This refers to the ability to perform various physical activities, such as endurance, strength, and flexibility, effectively and efficiently. Physical fitness is critical for maintaining good health, reducing the risk of chronic diseases, and improving quality of life.
- ❖ **Mental fitness:** This refers to the ability to manage stress, maintain a positive outlook, and make sound decisions. Mental fitness is important for maintaining overall well-being and reducing the risk of mental health issues.
- ❖ **Emotional Fitness:** This refers to the ability to manage emotions. To be more compassionate about life, nature, animals and other human beings. Emotional fitness is important for maintaining a great mental fitness and bring in positivity, love, compassion, care, attachment and a great connection with everything. And a

great connection always leads to a great level of fitness and Consciousness.

- ❖ **Nutrition:** A balanced and healthy diet is crucial for both physical and mental fitness. Eating a variety of nutrient-rich foods can help maintain energy levels, support healthy body composition, and reduce the risk of chronic diseases.
- ❖ **Rest and recovery:** Getting adequate rest and recovery time is important for both physical and mental fitness. Proper sleep and recovery can help the body and mind recharge, reduce the risk of injury, and improve overall performance.
- ❖ **Lifestyle factors**: This includes elements such as stress management, physical activity, and social support, which all play a role in maintaining overall physical and mental well-being.

The wise aspects of fitness recognize that physical, emotional and mental health are interconnected, and that a comprehensive approach to wellness involves attention to all these aspects, not just one or two. And that means you achieve fitness at 'Quantum Levels' and become **'Quantum Fit'**.

These wise aspects of fitness help us to get better understanding of our own body, our own self. We come to know what our strengths and weaknesses are. And the best part is that, with better understanding of our own self on physical level, psychological level, emotional level and spiritual Levels, we come to know, what are the areas of improvement. And we can act accordingly in regards to improve our own self on all levels of 'Fitness'.

By following a 'Quantum Fit' Lifestyle, we can see tremendous improvements in different aspects, like better functioning of the CNS (Central Nervous System)—improved mind-body or mind-muscle co-ordination; improved functional strength, performance, and improvement in day-to-day work; as well as accuracy and speed in routine work. Positive thinking, a positive approach, a positive mind-set Cultivating and maintaining good, healthy habits in our lifestyle Better connection with self, others, nature, and surroundings is possible because of improved sense and alertness, which are achieved through the great conditioning of the physical body through daily exercise and workout routines.

We receive good positive vibes all the time. Positivity right from the cell level. Improved communication and connectivity at cell level.

Improved exchange of gases, liquids and nutrition. Improved absorption of nutrition, oxygen and all essentials at cell level.

Improved functioning of all internal systems – including cardiovascular system, blood circulation, respiratory system, digestive system, reproductive system, central nervous system etc.

Maintained balance of different chemicals, fluids, liquids, water, salts, minerals, acids and alkali.

Energy balance.

Hormonal balance.

More production of required good hormones.

Removal of accumulated heavy metals, toxins, acids, chemicals, cellular debris and carcinogenic waste materials from the entire system.

Regularise metabolism at cell level.

Removal of excess fats accumulated and surrounded at different internal organs, muscles, vessels etc.

So apart from the commonly known aspects (visible or measurable) which are highlighted by most of the fitness professionals, there are many other aspects we may consider which might be at different and multiple levels like physical, psychological, emotional, spiritual, internal and external as well. And it may cover the dimensions at deepest, widest and tiniest levels of one's physical, physiological, body and surroundings and psychology, spiritual body and meta physical or holographic surroundings. And the response of one's body towards different situations, processes and connections might be different physically, physiologically, psychologically, emotionally, spiritually or meta physically. It's all about the interaction or give and take at cell level, physical level, psychological level, emotional level, spiritual level and universal level.

Sunlight has a direct effect on all living bodies in the nature. As most us must be knowing that sunlight is a combination of different colours. And these colour codes represent different nutritional values or contribute in activating and stimulating different minerals present inside the human, animal or any plant body. That's why sunlight have a great importance in achieving a great level of Fitness and Health.

So, make sure to spend ample of time under the sun, no matter at what time of the day, just expose your skin to the sun, **but without using sunscreen lotion or cream**.

Similarly spend time in fresh air, nature, alongside rivers, lakes, around trees, gardens, forest and farm etc. Air filled with plenty of **oxygen** is another important aspect which keeps us healthy.

Fresh, Clean and potable **pure water** from its original source is also an important factor to keep us in the healthiest state.

Everything around us carries certain frequencies, some sort of vibrations and which we can connect with, in the form of energy. Everything around us or everything we deal with in our day today life carries certain type and number of energies in the form of vibrations and frequencies, so it is very important to be wiser about the selection and choice we made to be surrounded with or get in connection with and be around with. We have choice to select what we want and what we don't.

"If you want to find the secrets of the universe, think in terms of energy, frequency and vibrations." – Nikola Tesla

Everything in this universe is about colours, vibrations, energies and frequencies, one need to connect or tune into right ones.

And all this is possible with constant efforts on a planned and trusted process of your fitness journey.

Type of Workouts commonly known

There are several types of workouts that one can engage in, depending on their goals, preferences, and fitness level. Some of the most common types of workouts include:

1. **Cardiovascular (Aerobic) Exercise:** This type of workout focuses on improving the health of the heart and lungs, and includes activities like running, cycling, swimming, and jumping rope. Cardiovascular exercise can help increase endurance, boost energy levels, and burn calories.

2. **Strength Training:** Strength training, also known as weightlifting, involves lifting weights or using resistance bands to build muscle and improve overall strength. This type of workout can help increase muscle mass, improve posture, and reduce the risk of injury.

3. **High-Intensity Interval Training (HIIT):** HIIT workouts are intense, short bursts of exercise interspersed with periods of rest. This type of workout can help improve cardiovascular fitness, boost metabolism, and burn more calories in a shorter amount of time.

4. **Yoga:** Yoga is a physical, mental, and spiritual practice that originated in ancient India. It involves a series of postures and breathing exercises designed to improve flexibility, strength, and balance. Yoga can also help reduce stress, improve sleep, and increase mindfulness.
5. **Pilates:** Pilates is a low-impact form of exercise that emphasizes controlled movements and correct posture. It was developed by Joseph Pilates in the early 20th century and is designed to improve flexibility, balance, and core strength.
6. **Bodyweight Training:** Bodyweight training involves using your own body weight as resistance to build strength and improve fitness. Examples of bodyweight exercises include push-ups, squats, and lunges. This type of workout is convenient because it can be done anywhere, without any equipment.
7. **Stretching and Flexibility Training:** Stretching and flexibility training involves holding a series of static stretches to increase flexibility and reduce muscle tension. This type of workout is important for maintaining good posture and reducing the risk of injury.

Each type of workout has its own unique benefits and can be incorporated into a comprehensive fitness routine to achieve a variety of health and wellness goals.

Wisely categorized types of Workouts

As we have understood, human body is most complex structure, similarly Human body responds differently for different exercises on an individual basis, that means same exercise could be different or give different effect on an individual, so there could be slight difference in the mechanism for different bodies depending upon many factors like Gender, Age, Medical Conditions or Physical limitations, physiology, genes, psychology, type of physical activity, it's speed and intensity etc. So, Exercises can be divided grossly into 2 types Aerobic and Anaerobic Exercises and this division is on technical basis but actually 'Aerobic' and 'Anaerobic' are the phases where body lands in to and adapts a specific mechanism for the time being depending upon multiple factors, majorly either because of actual intensity or speed of the workouts or condition and response of internal organs like Heart and Lungs of that particular person, further they can be divided into 5 types grossly, which are as follows:

1) **Aerobic Exercises:**

   Aerobic exercise is any type of cardiovascular conditioning. It can include activities like brisk walking, swimming, running, or cycling.

By definition, aerobic exercise means "with oxygen." Your breathing and heart rate will increase during aerobic activities.

Best Examples of Aerobic Exercises: Brisk Walk, Jogging, Dancing, Climbing Stairs or a Hill, playing any sport, swimming or even any physical activity or work like Digging, Gardening, Racking etc.

Even 'Circuit Training' with lowest weights and higher repetitions can be considered under 'Aerobic' type of exercises.

Importance of Aerobic Exercises:

Aerobics exercise helps to Increase stamina, Improves cardiovascular endurance conditioning.

Helps in better Conditioning of the Cardiac Muscles and Decreases risk of heart disease.

Helps to Lower blood pressure, only if done in moderate way and with regular practice and gradual progression.

Helps to better control blood sugar.

Assists in weight management and/or weight loss.

Improves lung function.

Decreases resting heart rate.

You might also have heard about 'Fat Burn Zone' theory, in which exercising at **around 60% to 70% of your maximum heart rate** will bring our bodies into a so-called "fat burning zone", optimal for losing weight. And it is also said that the Body fat is directly utilised as a source of Fuel to perform the Aerobic Activity, that means the fat is directly burned while doing the exercise, but the actual process of burning the fat begins only after first 20 Minutes of the actual start of the activity, but this time period might be different for different people, depending up on multiple factors like, body type, age, weight and so on. Also, you need to do for longer duration to achieve a good amount of fat burn, but compare to Increased BMR achieved by doing Strength Training, the calories burn would be very less.

(To Find out your maximum heart rate, subtract your age from 220. For example, a 35-year-old Person's maximum heart rate is 220 minus 35 — or 185 beats per minute. To enter the fat-burning zone, he/she'd want her heart rate to be **70 percent (ideal range is 60%-70%) of 185**, which is about **130** beats per minute. – **As I always say, one should not be very calculative, so just maintain the consistency, give your best and make sure that your workouts are safe and sustainable**)

2) Anaerobic Exercises:

Anaerobic exercise is any activity that breaks down glucose for energy without using oxygen. Generally, these activities are of short length with high intensity. The idea is that a lot of energy is released within a small period of time, and your oxygen demand surpasses the oxygen supply.

Example: Strength Training (To be more Specific, Progressive Weight Training in the Gym is the best Example of Strength Training).

Importance of Anaerobic Exercises:

Anaerobic exercise **helps boost metabolism as it builds and maintains lean muscle**. The leaner muscle you have, the more calories you'll burn during your next workout session. High-intensity exercise is also thought to increase your post-workout calorie burn, because Muscle is metabolically an active tissue, it requires calories to perform its own internal functions, so if you increase and maintain more muscles, naturally your BMR (Basal Metabolic Rate) would be High.

Increases bone strength and density. Anaerobic activity — like resistance training — can increase the strength and density of your bones.

1. Helps in weight maintenance.
2. Increases power and strength.
3. Regularise and Boosts metabolism.
4. Increases lactic threshold.
5. Reduces Stress, Fights depression.
6. Reduces risk of disease.
7. Protects joints.

3) **Stretches for Flexibility:**

Flexibility can be defined as the capacity of a joint or muscle to move through its full range of motion. And it could be achieved by following different flexibility exercises, some best-known examples are given below.

Examples: Stretches, Joint Mobility Drills and Yoga (Although Yoga is not Considered as an Exercise only, it's more about life style and it covers many aspects including Flexibility, Muscle Endurance, Core Strength, Breathing Exercises and So on).

Stretching doesn't fall under any category.

And stretches could be considered the major type under Flexibility.

Stretches can be divided further into 4 types, **Active stretching, Passive stretching,**

Dynamic stretching, and Proprioceptive Neuromuscular Facilitation (PNF) stretching.

PNF stands for Proprioceptive Neuromuscular Facilitation, which is a type of stretching that involves a combination of muscle contraction and relaxation, and passive and assisted stretching techniques. PNF stretches are often used in rehabilitation and physical therapy settings to improve range of motion, flexibility, and muscle strength.

There are several different techniques used in PNF stretching, but they all involve the following basic steps:

1. **Passive stretch:** The muscle group being stretched is placed in a stretched position, either by the individual or with the help of a partner or therapist.

2. **Isometric contraction:** The stretched muscle group is then contracted isometrically (without movement) against resistance for a short period of time (usually around 6 seconds).

3. **Relaxation:** The muscle group is then relaxed and allowed to return to its starting position.

4. **Passive stretch:** The muscle group is then stretched again, this time with greater ease due to the muscle's increased length and relaxation.

There are several variations of PNF stretching, including the hold-relax technique, the contract-relax technique, and the hold-relax-contract technique. Each variation has its own specific benefits and uses, but they all follow the basic steps outlined above.

PNF stretching is an effective way to improve flexibility and muscle strength, especially for athletes and individuals recovering from injury or surgery. However, it should be performed under the guidance of a trained professional to ensure safety and effectiveness.

And these different types of stretches could be used for different purposes and could be utilised at different stages of the workout flow.

The best example we can give for this is,

Dynamic stretches: Dynamic stretching is a movement-based type of stretching. It uses the muscles themselves to bring about a stretch. It's different from traditional "static" stretching because the stretch position is not held. And they are done at warm up or preparatory stage before the main workout. The purpose here to prepare and warm the body up for the next stage or next level of the workout.

Similarly,

Static Stretches: Static stretches are those in which you hold a single position for period of time, from 20 Seconds up to about 45 seconds, in a lying, seated or standing base position and target a particular or multiple muscle to stretch and relax them. The purpose here is to Relax the muscles completely down after the completion of main workout and to cooldown the body.

Importance of Flexibility Exercises:

Risk of injuries reduces drastically, as stiff muscles and least mobile joints are the main reason for most of the injuries.

Improved elasticity of Muscles.

Improved range of motion at joints.

Helps in conditioning of Joints, ligaments and muscles as well.

Reduces pain caused due to stiffness.

Improved Posture and Balance.

Supports most of the exercises and helps to improve the performance.

It's an important component in physical fitness.

It improves mobility, posture, muscle coordination.

It reduces the risk of intense muscle soreness.

4) **Balance:**

   Balance is the ability to control your body's position, whether stationary (i.e., a complex yoga pose) or while moving (e.g., skiing). **Balance** is a key component of **fitness**, along with strength, endurance, and flexibility.

   Example: Gymnastics, Roman Ring, Calisthenics and '**Mallakhamb**' (India's Famous Ancient Balance Exercise) etc.

   Importance of Balance Exercises:

   With practice, Improved coordination during balance training will be transferred into coordination in everyday life and improves day today life's overall performance by reducing risk factors.

   Helps in Joint Stability – Balance training stables multiple joints like spinal column, knees, ankles, hips, and shoulders.

Can prevent from risk of injuries including sprained ankles and serious knee problems or lower back issues.

5) Combination or Mixed Exercises:

This form of exercise is getting popular nowadays, because it covers almost all aspects or all types of exercises mentioned and is a combination of all or few of them.

And Functional Training, Cross Fit, Circuit Training etc. are the best examples of it.

A) Traditional Combination Workouts:

Practice/ Preparatory exercises like 'Dand' (Hindu Push-ups or Dive Bombs), 'Baithak' (Indian Style Body Weight Squats), Combination of 1 Dand and 1 'Baithak' simultaneously, called 'Sapatya' in Marathi language and few more similar exercises which are done as a part of preparation and regular practice for the Sport of 'Kushti' (Wrestling), which includes the perfect combination of Conditioning Exercises, Core strengthening, Strength, Stamina, Muscle Endurance, Balance and Flexibility.

Importance of Traditional Combination Exercises:

The human body is capable of multiple complex movements, by doing these types of exercises, movements improve and become more perfect.

1. Improved Performance and Movement Efficiency.
2. Improved Muscle Balance and Co-ordination.
3. Improved Muscle Endurance and Joint Mobility.
4. Increased Calorie Burn.
5. Improved Aerobic Capacity.
6. Improved Core Muscle engagement, performance and strength.

Traditional Combination Exercises use multiple joints and muscles. This type of training covers up all the aspects of fitness. It works on most of functional abilities of the body and with practice improves on them. Basic level, workouts Especially beneficial as part of a recovery or healing program in case of any injuries, especially in older adults to **improve balance – mind muscle co-ordination, agility and muscle strength**, and reduce the risk of falls.

B) 'Trending' Hybrid Combination Exercises:

HIIT (High Intensity Interval Training), Cross Fit, Functional Training, Circuit Training and Many more Trending Workout Combination patterns can be counted under this category. This type of activity is not for beginners.

Importance of Hybrid Combination Exercises:

All the benefits mentioned above in the Traditional Combination Exercises.

These exercises may be beneficial for the elite athletes, sports people or people doing exercises with right approach and having a conditioned body with great fitness levels. These workouts will help in improved performance in their sports or regular workouts.

But, over doing of anything might be harmful at times or if the person is not eligible/qualified (Not having good conditioned body and fitness levels), Especially while doing such Hybrid combination which requires fast movements, high impact movements, good mind muscle co-ordination or requires a great core muscles' strength and if any of the factor is lacking then it can be a big risk. Also, if the person's bones, joints and ligaments are not well conditioned or core muscles are not that much strong to have a good control on overall movements.

Every single sport and the practice (Specific or in general) to make the performance better, can be considered as a type of a complete 'Workout' in itself.

Here is a Small List (This list may include many more patterns and combinations of Workouts) of Combination of Workouts which includes and focus on different aspects of Fitness, like Strength, Stamina, Flexibility and Mobility of Joint and Muscles, Endurance, Core Strengthening, Stability, Balance and Overall Conditioning at various stages (Warm-up, Main Workouts and Cooldown) of the workouts.

Plyometrics:

It is a form of exercises that uses rapid movements to increase muscular power. Plyometrics, also known as jump training or plyos, are exercises in which muscles exert maximum force in short intervals of time, with the goal of increasing power. This training focuses on learning to move from a muscle extension to a contraction in a rapid or "explosive" manner, such as in specialized repeated jumping.

Calisthenics:

Calisthenics or callisthenics is a form of strength training consisting of a variety of movements that exercise large muscle groups, such as standing, grasping, pushing, etc. These exercises are often performed rhythmically and with minimal equipment, as bodyweight exercises.

The practice or art of Gymnastic exercises designed to develop muscular tone and promote physical well-being. Also, light gymnastics can be considered as the science, art, or practice of healthful exercise of the body and limbs, to promote strength, gracefulness, and general fitness; light gymnastics.

Functional Training:

Functional training can be explained as a sequel or combination of multiple exercises which involves training the body for the activities performed in daily life to improve overall Functional Strength of any person.

CrossFit:

CrossFit is a branded fitness regimen. This method was developed by Greg Glassman, who founded CrossFit with **Lauren Jenai** in **2000**, with CrossFit its registered trademark. It involves constantly varied functional movements performed at high intensity.

Cross Fit is a form of HIIT, set in a number of patterns and exercises included.

Circuit Training:

Circuit training is a form of body conditioning that involves endurance training, resistance training, high-intensity aerobics, and exercises performed in a circuit, similar to High-intensity interval training. It targets strength building and muscular endurance. Using it in an effective way, one can directly burn fat as a fuel in a circuit training format by maintaining heart rate into 'Fat Burn' zone.

Gymnastics:

Gymnastics is a type of sport that includes physical exercises requiring balance, strength, flexibility, agility, coordination, dedication and endurance.

The movements involved in gymnastics contribute to the engagement and development of the arms, legs, shoulders, back, chest, and abdominal muscle groups, most importantly the 'Core Muscles' group.

Kick Boxing Workouts:

Kickboxing is a close contact combat sport focused on kicking and punching. The combat takes place in a boxing ring, normally with boxing gloves, mouthguards, shorts, and bare feet to favour the use of kicks. Kickboxing is practiced for self-defences, general fitness, or for competition.

These workouts majorly focus on developing Strength in upper body, core muscle group as well as lower body. It Also focuses on increasing endurance (both cardiovascular and muscular), balance and quick reflexes etc. One needs to develop a great CNS functioning to actually perform in the competition.

Wrestling:

Wrestling is a series of combat sports involving grappling-type techniques such as clinch fighting, throws and takedowns, joint locks, pins and other grappling holds. Wrestling techniques have been incorporated into martial arts, combat sports and military systems.

Wrestling is played in different styles in different countries in the world. And out of it most ancient known and mentioned in Ancient Scriptures is in India. It is known as 'Kushti' in India. In India it is being played in Soil (Which is prepared especially by mixing different liquids and edible nutritious things, like some types of essential oils, ghee, butter, milk, curd etc. in the soil, preferably red coloured soil). But in modern days it's been played on the Mat, at competitive levels, nationally as well as internationally.

The exercises for the preparation, includes a great combination of Strength training, endurance training, mobility, conditioning, flexibility and it includes some of the Yoga Based practices as well.

Weight Training/ Weight lifting:

Weight training is a common type of strength training for developing the strength, size of skeletal muscles and maintenance of strength. It uses the force of gravity in the form of weighted bars, dumbbells or weight stacks, using weight training machines in order to oppose the force generated by muscle through concentric or eccentric contraction.

Weightlifting generally refers to activities in which people lift weights, often in the form of dumbbells or barbells. People lift various kinds of weights for a variety of different reasons.

Power Lifting:

Powerlifting is a strength sport that consists of three attempts at maximal weight on three lifts: squat, bench press, and deadlift. As in the sport of Olympic weightlifting, it involves the athlete attempting a maximal weight single-lift effort of a barbell loaded with weight plates.

Tai Chi:

Tai chi, short for Tai chi ch'üan, sometimes called "shadowboxing", is an internal Chinese martial art practiced for defence training, health benefits and meditation. Tai chi has practitioners worldwide from Asia to the Americas.

Many people practice Tai Chi to maintain their physical fitness.

Martial Arts:

Martial arts are codified systems and traditions of combat practiced for a number of reasons such as self-defence; military and law enforcement applications; competition; physical, mental, and spiritual development; entertainment; and the preservation of a nation's intangible cultural heritage.

Apart from the competitive levels, Martial Arts is practiced by many people around the worlds for Physical Fitness.

Tabata:

The Tabata Training method was originally created in Japan by a speed skating team head coach. The method was proven and named after a professor and researcher at the National Institute for Health and Nutrition. The Four Minute Workout promises to deliver a heart pumping, sweat inducing, super-fast paced HIIT workout.

Boot Camp:

A boot camp workout is basically a type of HIIT, bursts of intense activities alternated with intervals of lighter activity. A boot camp workout also can include functional fitness, such as using whole-body, multi-joint exercises that simulate movements people do in life.

Zumba: Zumba is a fitness program that involves cardio and Latin-inspired dance. It was founded by Colombian dancer and choreographer **Beto Pérez** in **2001**, and by 2012, it had 110,000 locations and 12 million people taking classes weekly. Zumba is a trademark owned by Zumba Fitness, LLC.

Aerobics:

Aerobics is a form of physical exercise that combines rhythmic aerobic exercise with stretching and strength training routines with the goal of improving all elements of fitness. It is usually performed to music and may be practiced in a group setting led by an instructor, although it can be done solo and without musical accompaniment.

Dance Exercise:

In dance, you achieve aerobic exercise by moving, jumping, and twirling. The anaerobic type of exercise comes when you hold positions like squatting and balancing. No matter the dance-whether it is tango, rumba, cha-cha, or waltz-you get both aerobic and anaerobic benefits.

Dance is a wonderful form of expression while also being a great way to work out and do some cardio while having fun. Dance is a universal practice with many different styles that have been practiced as long as history has been recorded. Whether you are a professional or just like to dance for fun, it is a great way to get yourself moving and build strength throughout your practice.

Skipping Rope:

A skipping rope or jump rope is a tool used in the sport of skipping/jump rope where one or more participants jump over a rope swung so that it passes under their feet and over their heads. There are multiple subsets of skipping/jump rope, including single freestyle, single speed, pairs, three-person speed, and three-person freestyle.

Many people do this as a whole workout.

Pilates:

Pilates (/ p ɪ ˈ l ɑː t iː z /; German: [piˈlaːtəs]) is a type of mind-body exercise developed in the **early 20th century** by **German** physical trainer **Joseph Pilates**, after whom it was named. Pilates called his method

"Contrology". It is practiced worldwide, especially in countries such as Australia, Canada, South Korea, the United States and the United Kingdom.

Pilates strengthens the thigh muscles (quadriceps), and this may help prevent arthritis and knee injuries. It may also help prevent greater disability if you have arthritis.

Power Yoga:

Power Yoga is any of several forms of energetic vinyasa-style yoga as exercise developed in America in the 1990s.

Basically, most of the poses and sequence of exercises developed in power yoga are derived from ancient form of Suryanamaskars and Yoga.

It is just an innovative form of traditional Yoga and Suryanamaskars' combination with few different variations.

Yoga:

Yoga is a group of physical, mental, and spiritual practices or disciplines which originated in ancient India and aim to control and still the mind, recognizing a detached witness-consciousness untouched by the mind and mundane suffering.

Surya Namaskar (Sun Salutation):

Surya Namaskar is the best example of ancient wisdom & knowledge about the human body. It comprises 12 steps that are purposefully woven together to benefit mind and body in various ways. Surya Namaskar is a practice in itself as well as a warming-up before performing further yoga asanas. It allows for "opening" of the body as it stretches, strengthens and lengthens all muscle groups. And in today's time, in the modern workouts like weight training exercises & HIIT workouts 'suryanamaskars' can be utilised effectively in the beginning of the workout, as preparatory exercises in the warm up part, and also can be used as a cooldown exercise focusing mainly on the stretching at the end part of the workout.

Meditation:

Meditation is a practice in which an individual uses a technique – such as mindfulness, or focusing the mind on a particular object, thought, or activity – to train attention and awareness, and achieve a mentally clear and emotionally calm and stable state. Meditation is practiced in numerous religious traditions. It is a great exercise for mind.

Meditation helps in having clarity of thoughts. It helps in improving on Mental Health and Fitness.

Pranayama:

'Pranayam' (also known as pranayama) is the ancient practice of controlling your breath in order to control the movement of life force ('Prana') through your body. Practicing pranayama is said to help calm and centre the mind while soothing the body. Pranayam can be done on its own or before, during, or after a series of yoga poses (asanas).

Pranayama is the yogic practice of focusing on breath. In Sanskrit, prana means "vital life force", and yama means to gain control. In yoga, breath is associated with prana, thus, pranayama is a means to elevate the prana shakti, or life energies. Pranayama is described in Hindu texts such as the Bhagavad Gita and the Yoga Sutras of Patanjali.

Running:

Running is a method of terrestrial locomotion allowing humans and other animals to move rapidly on foot. Running is a type of gait characterized by an aerial phase in which all feet are above the ground. And could be used as an effective form of exercise or workout to maintain a good physical fitness.

Many people consider and do it as a whole workout.

Jogging:

Jogging is a form of trotting or running at a slow or leisurely pace. The main intention is to increase physical fitness with less stress on the body than from faster running but more than walking, or to maintain a steady speed for longer periods of time. Performed over long distances, it is a form of aerobic endurance training.

Walking:

Walking is one of the main gaits of terrestrial locomotion among legged animals. Walking is typically slower than running and other gaits. Walking is defined by an 'inverted pendulum' gait in which the body vaults over the stiff limb or limbs with each step. This applies regardless of the usable number of limbs walk.

For some people walking few meters or kilometres could possibly be their 'Whole Workout'.

Brisk Walk:

A brisk walk is a form of physical activity that involves walking at a faster pace than usual, typically at a pace of 3.5 to 4.5 miles per hour (5.6 to 7.2 kilometres per hour). It is a moderate-intensity aerobic activity that can help to improve cardiovascular health, increase energy levels, and promote weight loss.

Brisk walking is a low-impact exercise that can be done almost anywhere, at any time, and does not require any special equipment or gym membership. It is a simple and effective way to incorporate physical activity into your daily routine, and can be easily adapted to your fitness level and personal preferences.

To achieve a brisk walking pace, aim to take longer strides and swing your arms as you walk. You should also breathe deeply and evenly, maintaining a comfortable but slightly elevated heart rate throughout your walk. A typical brisk walk can last anywhere from 30 minutes to an hour, depending on your schedule and fitness goals.

Overall, brisk walking is a safe and effective way to improve your health and well-being, and is a great form of exercise for people of all ages and fitness levels.

Trekking:

Trekking can be done solo or as a group, and it usually entails walking on some form of trail (like a trail hike) for an extended period of time. It's an activity that is typically done for enjoyment, exercise, or exploration. Trekking is different from other types of hiking because you are not required to carry heavy backpacks to camp.

Hiking:

Hiking is a long, vigorous walk, usually on trails or footpaths in the countryside. Walking for pleasure developed in Europe during the eighteenth century. Religious pilgrimages have existed much longer but they involve walking long distances for a spiritual purpose associated with specific religions.

Swimming:

Swimming is the self-propulsion of a person through water, or other liquid, usually for recreation, sport, exercise, or survival. Locomotion is achieved through coordinated movement of the limbs and the body to achieve hydrodynamic thrust which results in directional motion.

Many people do Swimming as their 'Whole Workout'.

And each type of workout mentioned above can be considered as **'unique in its own way'**.

Most of the Sports and their practices also considered as a specific type or unique in its own way.

There is a great variety and different way to maintain **'Physical Fitness'**, but the **'Wise Choice'** is yours. Always!!

General Sequence of Workouts

The sequence and flow of workouts or exercises refers to the order in which exercises are performed and the progression from one exercise to the next. It is an important factor in determining the effectiveness of a workout and reducing the risk of injury.

Typically, a workout starts with a warm-up to raise the heart rate and prepare the body for exercise. This could involve light cardio or dynamic stretching.

Next, the main workout is usually structured in a specific sequence to target specific muscle groups or to improve specific fitness components, such as strength, endurance, or flexibility. This typically includes a combination of resistance training exercises for specific muscle groups, such as weights or bodyweight exercises, as well as cardio exercises to improve cardiovascular fitness.

The order of exercises within a workout can vary, but there are certain guidelines that are commonly followed to optimize results. For example, large muscle groups such as the legs and back are usually targeted first, while smaller muscle groups like the arms and shoulders are worked on later in the workout. Compound exercises, which target multiple muscle groups at once, are usually performed before isolation exercises, which target individual muscles.

After the main workout, a cool-down period is usually included to bring the heart rate back to normal and help the body recover. This could involve light cardio or static stretching.

The sequence and flow of a workout is a carefully planned and structured process that helps to optimize results and reduce the risk of injury, and that's why it is very important to take advice from a Certified and Experienced Fitness expert in regards to your workout programming.

General Sequence and Flow of Exercises:

Generally, People, follow this (as mentioned below) sequence.

Warm up – Main Workout – Post workout Stretches.

But ideally, they should follow this sequence which is mentioned below, in details.

Warm-up:

Actually, this concept could be different for different people. Suppose, if 'Running' is considered as the main workout on a cardio day for someone then at the same time the same exercise of 'Running' could be just a warmup for someone else as a part of their workout.

This Normally includes Any form of cardio (Walking, Running, Indoor Cardio Exercises, Walk on Treadmill, Stationary Cycle, Outdoor Cycling and many more options for 5 to 10 Minutes). And this warm up may be different for Cardio based workouts, Strength Workouts, Flexibility and Balance workouts like Yoga, Power Yoga, Pilates etc. or for any sports workout routine.

There might be different patterns of warm up or different stages as per the requirement or as per the type of workouts or as per the muscles and joints' involvement. So, we may further divide it in to different stages. Or we may just consider these as different stages from different intensity levels. Some people may follow or may not follow any particular flow or sequence of warm up stages or patterns as per the need or requirements of their workout routine. They might do as per their understandings. There are no fixed criteria as such. And there is a free will, always.

A) **General Warm up for the Entire body**: Which includes Joint Mobility Drills and this includes different type of movements like Rotations, Circular Movements, Semi Circular movements or Half circles, Twisting, bending, Flexions, Extensions, Elevations, Depressions,

Protractions, Retractions and so on depending on the type of joints and its range of motion as per the current body condition, Fitness level, Body structure, Body symmetry, Body posture, Ratio of Muscle balance and coordination in between opposite (Agonist/Antagonist) Muscles, Limitations (if any) as per medical conditions or injuries or postural defects or structural changes. Plus, there might be some add on to general mobility drills to look after specific areas or joints or muscles as per the specific medical condition, injury or body limitations or lifestyle structural defect or pain or to bring in the proper muscle balance or to strengthen the weak muscles.

In Full Body warm up, we are actually supposed to first start with joint mobility drills for all the major joints of the body right from Neck, Shoulders, Elbows, Wrists, Spine, Hip Joint, Knees, Ankles etc. These Mobility drills are supposed to be done is a slow, steady, controlled and rhythmic manner and are never supposed to do very fast, impactful, jerky or uncontrolled movements. We should do the movements or complete the range of motion as per one's body limitations and in the comfort zone, never ever push too hard in the beginning itself. It's kind of waking up the body especially when you are working out in the Morning time, after a sleep of 6-8 Hrs. So, it becomes very necessary to wake/activate the muscles, joints, entire body slowly and prepare for a basic, moderate or intense workout. Obviously, it makes sense to start with a wise sequence and then reach up to the peak in a systematic and planned way. In the routine of Yoga, these are called, 'Sukshma Vyayam' and there is no specific sequence given, some people do it in the beginning, some people do it in between or by the end of the Yoga Asan Practices. But if we are looking for weight training specifically then these micromovements or joint mobility drills are supposed to be done in the beginning itself. Also, the sequence of joint doesn't matter much, some people start with Neck & some may start with ankle joint, there is no ideal sequence as such.

B) **Cardio as a Warm up**: There are two Major Types of Cardio Exercises which we may consider as a Good Warm up. They are as follows –

  1) **Indoor Cardio**: It can be further divided into 2 types –

     a) **Freehand Exercises** (Different types or Combination of variety of exercises using own body weight or some props Depending up on the intensity levels considering availability of space and props, body type, BMI and physical limitation etc).

It may include Spot Walking, Spot Marching, Spot Jogging, Spot Running, Skipping, Jumping Jacks, Mountain Climbers, Burpees, Suryanamaskars (Fast Pace) and combination of few or all of above-mentioned exercises, it completely depends on the person doing it and as per the situation.

b) **Cardio Machine Exercises**: It may include Cardio equipment available at home, commercial gym, office gym or club house etc.

Exercises like Walking, Sprinting, Running, Jogging, Interval training or any specific inbuilt program designed in the machine itself, on a Tread Mill.

Similarly, cycling (with low resistance and high speed or with high resistance and low speed – depending up on the individuals doing the exercise) on a stationary bike or spinning bike etc.

And there are few more cardio machines designed which works more effectively than the normal Treadmill or a cycle, we may count on Cross trainer, Elliptical, Climb Mill or step climber, Rowing machine etc and so on, plus nowadays there are Ski-ergs, Air Bike, Arc Trainer, Versa Climber, Manual Treadmill (Treadmill without Motor), Curve Treadmills etc and so on.

c) **Specific type Warm up as per the requirement of Group Classes**: These type of Group activities including Aerobics, Zumba, Dance Exercises, Kick Boxing, Circuit Training and some of the HIIT Classes like Cross fit, Functional Training etc.

But in case, as a part of a short warm up, we cannot consider the entire routine of this. We may consider few basic steps for a limited period of time of 5 to 10 Minutes as a Good Warm up.

2) **Outdoor Cardio**: There are Variety of Exercises which can be done outdoor.

First thing which I would like to mention is that, all the indoor body weight exercises can be done outdoor as well, all the group classes also can be done outdoor. Plus, most of the outdoor sports can be considered as the outdoor cardio or combination workouts.

Exercises like outdoor walk (slow, moderate, fast speed) brisk walk, jogging, Marching, running (Slow, moderate, fast speed), sprints, long distance low pace running, climbing up hill, steps, outdoor cycling, swimming (apart from rivers, wells, lakes, beaches, back waters, can be done in outdoor and indoor pools as well), trekking etc.

But if we consider just the part of warm up then a good brisk walk, running, step climbing or walking up the hill, cycling etc could be the best options.

Here also the same principle could be applicable for all i.e., if a particular outdoor activity might be warmup for a person and the same activity with same intensity might possibly be the main workout for another person. Again, it depends upon multiple factors.

C) **Local Area Warmup/ Specific Body Part/ Specific Muscles or Group of Muscles**: This type of warm up is majorly done on strength training day. It is also called as 'Local Muscle Warm up'. People after completing the general warm up and before starting the main workouts, generally do it for the preparation of high intensity workout sets of that particular Muscle or group of Muscles. For example, if someone is going to do Upper Body workouts, he/she might do Push-up or Pull ups or Hindu Push ups as a Local warm up in order to do further main workouts of upper body. And to be more specific on intensity levels someone might do easy variations of upper body workouts to start with and to prepare for the main workouts, for example: someone who's main workout is of back muscles, then he/she might start with Mid/Seated Row Machine or Lat Pull Down Machine, with low to moderate weight and a greater number of repetitions in order to bring in more blood circulation in the targeted area for enhanced performance in the main sets.

Importance of warm-up:

- If we start with a wise and sensible choice of required exercises in a systematic way, then this will be a good warm up and it can lead to the most effective and satisfactory experience of the main workout with full safety of muscles, ligaments, joints and internal organs.

Warming up is really very important. Now let's, understand the benefits of all the stages in the warm-up part.

Let's talk about the 1st stage of warm up i.e., 'Basic Joint Mobility Drills', by following these drills we actually try to wake the entire body, up.

We try to activate the Muscles and Joints which we are going to use in the Main Workouts.

It helps in increased range of motion in between joints, we may call it as Mobility or Flexibility.

Increased Viscosity of Synovial Fluid in the Joints to make the joints work more smoothly and create safer environment for the Bones, Joints and Ligaments to function effectively.

Improved sensitivity of CNS receptors.

Let's Know the Benefits of 2nd stage of Warm up i.e., Cardio as a 'Warm up'. Moderate intensity Cardio as a warm-up can be considered a good choice to start with. Here are the good points about the Cardio in the warm up –

A Cardio warm up is supposed to be done for the time duration in between 5 Minutes to 10 Minutes.

It actually Increases Blood Circulation in Entire Body especially more in the lower body, and it is a good warm up on the Lower Body's workout day.

It raises the body temperature up to a certain required level, which is a kind of preparation for safe Main Workouts.

Increases heart rate up to necessary levels for the main workouts.

Increases the oxygen supply.

In short it helps to stimulate and activate cardiovascular system as well as respiratory system.

Preparing the body for the higher intensity workouts which you are supposed to do in the main workouts.

Improved Mind – Muscle Co-ordination.

Let's know the Benefits of 3rd stage of warm up (Body flow like Surya Namaskar or a Body Flow Power Yoga Circuit or World's Greatest stretch or any other specific stretches or drills or Dynamic Stretching or any particular movement or exercise etc)

In the above mentioned all the stretches and in all possible formats (Dynamic, Active or Static or Slow tempo) The major benefits are to improve Flexibility, Mobility and Activation of all the Important but most of the time ignored, Internal Minor Muscles or Major Muscles or Group of Muscles of the following joints or Group of Joints – Entire Spinal Column (Deep as well as superficial Muscles present in Cervical, Thoracic, Lumber etc.), Shoulder Joints (Rotator Cuff Muscles), Hip Joints (Gluteus Group) and Core Muscle Group.

It Improves Concentration due to improved CNS (Central Nervous System) Functionality.

Improves alertness and reduces response time, so better connection with surroundings and environment, more awareness about the situation and accordingly wise and sensible decision making in any work or in the workouts, basically more focus on the target muscles or area.

Balance and Proper deviation of Energy equally throughout the entire body or more towards the working muscles or body parts.

Improved blood circulation in the above-mentioned joints and muscle groups.

Reduced risk of injuries, due to proper warm up, mobility, focus and stability.

Accelerates your performance in the main workouts.

Gives proper balance, full range of motion and a firm ground stability in all main workouts (which could be the optimum utilization of your energies, strengths and stamina or endurance etc.)

- **One should do, daily once or twice a sequence of Micro movements covering all of the joints right from head to toe, to maintain a great conditioning of their joint health.**

- In warm up, some people just do Body Flow or Joint Mobility drills from Head to toe for all the joints. Some people just do certain specific movements or Multi joint movements to activate few muscles or group of muscles and the major focus could be on Core Muscles. If we consider a Good Body Flow, focusing on major muscles and core muscles then starting with Basic Joint Mobility or 'Sukshma Vyayam' one can do 'Surya Namaskars' or 'World's Greatest Stretch' or the Basic Body flow in 'Power Yoga', as per the demand or requirement of that specific workout on that particular day. And this can be called as a Second stage or level in the sequence of Warm-up.

- Some people consider Only a Moderate intensity Cardio as a Warm-up. And then they directly start with their main workouts. Especially on Weight Training Days.

- Some people do both Joint Mobility Drill and Cardio and then do their Main Workouts.

- Some people do Joint Mobility Drills (Sukshma Vyayam) then Cardio (Brisk Walk, Running or any Cardio Machine) then 2nd stage of warm up (Body flow like Surya Namaskar or a Body Flow Power Yoga Circuit or World's Greatest stretch or any other specific stretches or drills or Dynamic Stretching or any particular movement or exercise etc) as per the requirement of the main workouts they are going to do at that time.

- Some people don't even do cardio or any kind of joint mobility drills or 'body flow' or any specific stretches, they directly start with moderate weight 'Local Muscle Warm up' (Most of the people in this category don't even know that they are doing this, they consider this as their 1st set of their workout, but considering the choice of weight we may assume it as 'Local Muscle Warm-up'). Generally, they start with any Compound Exercise to target any specific major Muscle like Chest or Back.

But this might come with a risk of injury or We may call it as a 'Not very Safe' way to start with their workouts.

- Even we may see people starting with different sequences for example,

Some people may follow this sequence: 'Joint Mobility Drills' (Sukshma Vyayam) > 2nd stage of warm up (Body flow like Surya Namaskar or a Body Flow 'Power Yoga Circuit' or World's Greatest stretch or any other specific stretches or drills or Dynamic Stretching or any particular movement or exercise etc. there are multiple options, so different people different choices) > Moderate Intensity Cardio (Brisk Walk, Running or any Cardio Machine etc) > And then follow the further routine.

Some people may follow this sequence: Moderate Intensity Cardio (Brisk Walk, Running or any Cardio Machine etc) > 'Joint Mobility Drills' (Sukshma Vyayam) > 2nd stage of warm up (Body flow like Surya Namaskar or a Body Flow Power Yoga Circuit or World's Greatest stretch or any other specific stretches or drills or Dynamic Stretching or any particular movement or exercise etc) > And then further routine.

Some people may follow any one sequence or they might just do any 1 or 2 of the above mentioned by any flow or sequence as per their understanding and as per the habit of their workout routine.

In case if you have any, 'Body Limitations' or 'Physical Injury' or any 'Postural Change/Defect' because of the lifestyle or workstyle or any other reason, you should always follow the guidelines given by your doctor or Physiotherapist or any Qualified and Experienced Fitness Expert. Then the Physiotherapy Exercises can be prescribed and

included before warm up or after warm up and before main workouts as per the require recovery program. Also, there might be few exercises or movements or stretches which could be restricted which may aggravate the injury or pain or which should not be suiting to the recovery routine given by the Physiotherapist. So always follow the DO's and Don'ts list and as per the given sequence.

If you practice regularly, anything can be accepted and adapted by your body over the period of time. And that can actually work for you. Your body adapts it over the period of time. But 'Safety' should be the first priority, if you are looking for a sustainable and effective way of workouts or a fitness routine.

And the Most Important thing about the Warm-up is that, this routine or pattern of Warm up may change, as per the Intensity levels of the main workouts or Achieved fitness levels or the type of the workout or even as per the target muscle or group of muscles and even it might be different for sports, different for Strength Workouts, different for Cardio based and Floor Exercises, different for Yoga or Power Yoga and so on. It can be customised (For Personal Training or Rehab exercises Or Special Population as per the Requirement of the workout or as per the intensity levels or Fitness level or as per the physical limitations or as per the specific target/goal of the person etc) as well as In general (For a Group Class Or for any specific sports or General Warm-up but again there might be difference as per the type of Group class or Sports or the intensity Levels of the class, whether it's for Beginners, Intermediate Level or Advance Level etc). And this may change over the period of time with practice after achieving certain fitness levels or as per the Genuine requirement of the workout or body limitations or for the conditioning, consistency and so on. And even at sometimes just for a 'Change'.

I have seen people, who take shower with cold or room temperature water to increase the blood circulation before starting their workouts and they consider it as a Good General Warm up for the entire body.

Again, the same principle come into picture, Different People, Different Thoughts – Different Assumptions – Different Views – Different Choices and so it is.

Activation /Conditioning:

Activation of the muscle or group of muscles is to create warmth with proper blood circulation in that muscle, which further makes it more flexible and mobile as compared to a stiff or cold body. Basically, it is done by starting with gentle or mild movements with further progression which prepares these important parts for the next level of workouts where these muscles play an important role to make the workout more effective and keeping the surrounded joints, ligaments, minor muscles, deep muscles, tendons safer.

The main purpose of this is to increase the blood circulation in the Target Muscles as well as supporting muscles. More the Blood Circulation, more the nutrition and oxygen supplied and which leads to improved efficiency in the activity or the exercise and faster recovery.

This might be related to core muscles or some specific joints which will be utilised in the main workouts. So, it depends on what type of workouts will be there in the main workouts and which muscles will be targeted. So, the conditioning and Activation of all targeted muscles or and the supporting muscles which will be engaged in supporting the major muscles for balancing or to give stability in any particular action which is the part of the exercise or workout and that's why strengthening or conditioning or preparation of the supporting muscles or core muscles or some internal/deep muscles which holds the joints and makes the movements in main workouts possible in the safest and effective way. And this is very important.

This Activation and Conditioning Includes:

Balance out the opposite muscles: With regular practice to work on agonist and antagonist muscles one can have a great balance in between opposite muscles as per the proportion wise division. This principle is very helpful and effective in the compound movements, especially doing high intensity workouts. For example – Flat bench press – to make this more effective & lift maximum weight in the set, you will have to activate the rotator cuff muscles first with low intensity & high reps, then from this particular point of view of opposite muscles you are also supposed to do a couple of sets of static hold position of the lats' muscles to have more blood flow over there. Or just do a couple of sets of Lat pull down or mid row machine with static hold in the last repetition to activate these muscles, so that while actually doing the heavy main set of the bench press these muscles of back will remain firm by pressing on the bench in scapula retracted position in its' contracted position intact (as the first power generating point) to give a firm stability of back muscles (which is the requirement of the set) along with the other core muscles. Additionally, you may activate the lower back muscles (to have a firm grip by pressing the hips in the bench as the second power generating point in order to maintain the arch in the lumber area) as well and furthermore, a slight activation of hamstrings (to have a firmer grip by pressing the heels on the floor as the third power generating point) which will support and make the movement more effective & generate more power. And balance out the opposite muscles.

Effective Mobility of Joints – Range of motion of a joint depends on few factors, one of the most important factors is elasticity or flexibility of muscles which hold the joint. As we say stronger the muscles safer the joint, similarly we can also say greater the flexibility or elasticity safest the joint. Because flexible muscles or overall joint can easily absorb the sudden impact at any particular joint and reduce the risk of injury. Only strong and bulk of muscles could lead to risk of injury if the muscles are not flexible enough, because at the time of sudden accident or impact the stiff bulky muscles can worsen the situation than safeguarding the joint and ligaments.

One can improve mobility and flexibility by doing –

Joint mobility drills in warm up, on a regular basis.

Post workout stretches. Could be done actively or passively (With another person's help) or dynamically.

Yoga Poses (Yogasanas) on a regular basis.

(Know that, yoga is supposed to be done like yoga itself, that means it should never be done like an exercise where you are sweating, your heart beat is increasing, body temperature rising, increased blood circulation in overall body and unnecessary involvement or engagement of different other muscles those are not the targeted muscles. Or you feel very uncomfortable or feel pain while doing any stretch or a particular pose. And if you see these symptoms while doing any yoga pose then, just stop. Everything should be done with ease, comfort and within limit in yogic practices. Go with the flow as per your unique body design. Don't rush for anything. Observe, analyse and know your limits and act accordingly.)

While doing Stretches one should practice deep breathing and focus more on complete exhalation. To have a great control on breathing also, in order to calm the mind down, you may practice to observe the 'gap' in between the exhalation & inhalation. This is a great and most effective way, try it.

Active and dynamic stretching of muscles and joints which improves elasticity of the muscles further, leads to improved range of motion. So that target muscle's or group of muscles', involvement increases and the set of exercise or overall workout becomes more effective.

Strengthening of ligaments, tendons and muscles that means, overall strengthening and conditioning of the entire joint involved. This is important especially for the most delicate joints like Shoulder and Hip joints, because these joints are able to do almost 360-degree rotation and way more complex and can create trouble for rest of the body either upper body or lower body. These joints are bigger joint and are connected to multiple different muscles which includes superficial muscles as well as small internal/deep muscles which connects holds or gives stability or support in the motion at any particular angle or direction, to these joints. As both of these joints fall into ball and socket category and which covers a large range of motion and it can become quite risky at times if the load is way beyond the capacity of the person. And muscles attached or holding the joints are strong enough to lift the load but very stiff and in other situation if the internal/deep minor muscles which are holding the joint have been always neglected and become weak without conditioning over the period of time, could lead to risk of injury.

One should focus on balancing and coordination in between opposite muscles or in the same muscle group. And conditioning, of the muscles which surrounds and holds the joint together. Focus on, to increase flexibility and endurance and strength of all internal/deep minor muscles as well as superficial major muscles to make the movements more efficient, safe and effective. The more you practice and try to condition the body, the quality of movement and control on it increases further more.

In most of the cases those who work out regularly, the injuries may occur due to Sudden impact, may be because of an accident or overload while working out.

In some cases, the injuries might happen because of starting newly or restarting after a long gap, with incorrect workout program which doesn't suit as per one's current fitness levels and internal body conditioning. Where the intensity or the type of workout don't match with the current fitness levels and body condition.

Core Activation is necessary before any structural workouts like Deadlift or Squats. Core conditioning and strengthening is considered as a key factor, because these core muscles play an important role in most of the exercises.

Now let's understand what are core muscles and why they are so important?

Core Muscles includes Abdomen (Stomach) muscles, Oblique (Sides) muscles, Lower back muscles and some part of Glutes (Hips) muscles. As we see the structure of the human body, the upper extremity (upper body) and the lower extremity (lower body) connects at this point where these core muscles are surrounded. And there is no hard and bony structure which support this area, there is only spinal column getting attached to hip joint, that's why the muscles which surrounds this area becomes very important. This area is vital, because there are multiple important internal organs which are delicate and play an important role in physiological and biological functions of the human body. And these vital internal organs have to be protected all the time especially if the body is in action or performing any physical work or attempting any movement. Whenever body is in action and performing any free movement as simple as walking, these are the muscles which gets engaged first to support the movement and provide stability to balance and carry forward the movement or activity. And that's why strengthening, flexibility and proper conditioning of these core muscles is very important. If the movements are difficult or more intense and required more balancing or if the movements are impactful then, overall requirement of conditioning is more especially while doing workouts like, functional training or CrossFit or running etc. Otherwise, the risk of injuries can be considered more if the person is having weak core.

Another important reason why, people should start with core muscles conditioning first, before starting any workout routine is that, core muscles area or the trunk area gets affected mostly if the person is not working out for a long duration of time. Especially those people who have a Desk job or living a sedentary lifestyle, there are high chances that their core muscles become weaker day by day. First of all, because of lack of movement, the blood circulation towards core muscles decreases drastically, they become weak day by day, muscle loss happens due to which natural tightness and the tone in the stomach because of muscles reduces a lot, then because of lack of flexibility and mobility these muscles become stiff, and still if the person continued same lifestyle, then the actual structural changes in the spine might occur, like APT (Anterior pelvic tilt) and which might lead to Spondylitis or Herniated Disc or Disc Bulge at lumber region. And even the Transverse abdomen muscle due to weakness and loosening, can get tore at different locations because of sudden impact or load and may lead to Hernia. There are 7 types of Hernia and the root cause of all types is the weak core muscles and excessive visceral fat, which push the internal organs towards the stomach wall. There are 80% chances for Men to get Hernia compared to women and apart from just weak core muscles, there could be multiple reasons for this. Visceral Fat deposition increases, that means fat percentage increases in the stomach area in between the cavity of the stomach especially at the surroundings of the internal organs and outer layer and more at the lower part of the abdomen, this is the area where fat deposition starts very first and after a good exercise and diet routine with proper progression in all possible aspects, when fat loss happens and a good amount of fat percentage is dropped due to great conditioning of core muscles then at the last, the fat of this area decreases and one can see the actual visible changes, as well as inch loss happened.

Conditioning, strengthening and mobility exercises can be given in general for overall body and anybody can do if they don't have any injuries or medical conditions in specific.

And also, it can be customised as per the requirement or need on an individual level.

Rehab Exercise:

Includes, mobility of Joints, Active Stretching – Due to injury or over stiffness or weakness of certain superficial muscles or internal or deep muscles or overall stiffness in any particular joint due to different reasons, requires specific attention on a regular basis and specifically before the exercises where these muscles or joints are going to be utilised. To make the workouts safer for those specific muscles or joint affected and efficiently carry out the movements without any interruption due to pain or discomfort. With improved flexibility by regular practice, utilisation of more area of muscles can lead to good blood circulation and this will aid to fast recovery of that particular muscle or group of muscles or joint and bring it back to normal condition over the period of time. But the time required for a partial or full recovery from the injury might be depending up on multiple factors and as per the situation and individuals.

Strengthening of Ligaments, Tendons and Muscles.

Flexibility or Elasticity of Muscles.

Specific warm up or preparatory set or special preparation before starting with the exercises of a specific muscle, group of muscles or joint. For example,

A person with Knee Pain, can start with Light or moderate Weight Leg Extension Exercise on Machine before Weighted Squats or Leg Press Machine as a Main Compound Exercise in Lower body workout routine, to activate Quadriceps Muscles which safeguards the knee joint and reduce the pain due to increased blood supply in the knee joint while performing the main workouts.

All these points mentioned above are as per the requirement to rehab any particular Joint/ Muscle/ Tendon/Ligament etc.

In some cases, both or any of the above Steps Conditioning and Rehab Exercises can be required depending up on requirement of the case and other multiple factors.

The recovery period by rehab exercises completely depends on individual body's response to the set of exercises recommended by an expert and few other factors like age, lifestyle and so on.

Main Workouts:

The concept of the main workout in common is to do an intense work-out and get exhausted or get the satisfaction of burning maximum calories or pumping up the target muscles at its' maximum capacity. Most of the time, it is a kind of, state of mind, which could be illusion at some extent, where the body gets exhausted, muscles get pumped out completely and to achieve further contraction of specific muscle or group of targeted muscles after spending sufficient time or after doing specific number of sets of different exercises with maximum weight/poundage. By the end of the main workouts people get exhausted completely, they use their full energy and become too tired.

Main Workouts can be of different forms for different people, depending on multiple factors. Considering one's Age, Gender, Body type, as per the availability of the equipment or space (the Nature or Type of Main Workouts will depend on this specific point, whether the person should do Body Weight Exercises or using some equipment or machines, Outdoor or Indoor etc). Specific Fitness Goal (if any), Physical Limitations (if any), Medical Condition (if any), Injuries (if any), but the most important criteria should be Fitness Level, that means an experienced Coach can design the best suitable main workout for their client, considering their current fitness level and past fitness history and depending up on many other important factors.

In many cases, people consider the Main Workout is the only workout they are supposed and willing to do and they underestimate the warm up and cooldown part, which actually are the most important parts of anyone's workout routine, many people skip these parts and the basic concept of 'Complete Workout' doesn't get fulfilled.

The first thing is, by underestimating or skipping or by just doing as a formality, for the sake of doing or incomplete warm up and cooldown or by not doing what exactly is required in the warm up and cooldown as per the individual requirements. But, this is very important to understand what are the strengths and weaknesses on an individual basis and accordingly one should plan their warmup and cooldown routine as per the current conditioning of the body. For example, if anyone is having a stiff lower back and glute muscle then the person should include the mobility, conditioning drills and stretches for those specific muscles as well as joints to increase the mobility of joints, elasticity of interconnected muscles and endurance of the muscles.

In Main Workouts, we may consider the following sequence or flow of exercises in the routine.

Again, it may be different from person to person and as per the Fitness Levels.

Let's consider **Beginner Level** and understand who falls into this category. Those people who have never done the workouts before or those people who have done the workouts in past but there is a big gap and they are restarting the workouts.

The main workout for Beginner covers full body Muscles,

- Targeting Bigger Muscles initially and including exercises for them rather than targeting the supporting or smaller muscles specifically.

- Starting with Multi joint or Compound movements rather than single joint or concentration movements.

- Depending up on the facilities (Indoor/Outdoor).

- With or Without equipment or props or machines.

- If in a Gym, Preferably Supported, on Weight Training Machines.

- Starting with Major Muscles' exercises in Upper extremity (Chest, Back, Shoulders and Arms) and Lower extremity (Hips/Glutes, Thighs and Calf Muscles).

- Low to Moderate and slightly challenging intensity and less number of exercises per major muscle group.

- If the person is doing the workouts very first time in their life, then initially up to 1st two weeks there have to be 1 set per exercise and up to 10 Repetition for each set of exercise. And the intensity has to be Minimum to Average depending up on multiple factors like the Targeted Muscle, Type of Exercise, Age of the Person, Medical Condition or Injury or Physical Limitation, availability of equipment/ machines/props, choice or options of the exercise and so on.

- With consistency, further progression will be increased Number of repetitions up to 20 per set and increased number of sets up to 2 and if the person feels comfortable up to 3 Sets majorly.

- Consider 1st set as a Preparatory set, 2nd Set will be considered as Main Set with increased intensity and 3rd set will be final set where fullest capacity is challenged by maximum intensity for a specific repetition range. In some cases, people might do 4 or more sets as well, all depending up on the strategy of the designed workouts or the coach may take random decision on the spot as per the situation depending on many factors.

- Generally, after warm up and conditioning exercises the very 1st Exercise of strength training may have more than 3 sets if required, also when we change the muscle group, then also very 1st exercise might have more than 3 sets.

- In some cases, people may start with single joint movements or concentration movements followed by compound or multi joint movements or structural movements, depending up on the strategy of the workout program and free thoughts of the Fitness Coach who designed the workout program. The flow or the sequence of the workouts may be different for different people as per situation.

- Depending up on few of the factors like individual body's response (Positive/Negative) to the particular workout, speed of recovery and so on.

- Focus on improving the quality of the movements which includes slow, steady and controlled speed which is involved in different exercises, Range of Motion, Core Muscle Engagement, Mind Muscle Co-ordination and breathing techniques which may depend up on multiple factors like Age, type of exercise, intensity of workouts, medical conditions (if any) and so on.

People who are doing the workouts from quite some time, let's assume from past 3 to 6 Months and those who are doing their workouts with consistency and successfully progressed in the beginners' workouts in terms of Strength, Stamina, flexibility, quality of the movements in the exercises and so on, they fall in to Intermediate Level.

Again, the design or pattern of the workouts depends up on individual level progress, strengths, weaknesses (Medical Condition, Physical limitations, injuries etc), fitness goal or target, response of the body towards previous pattern of workout which he/she has done in past, availability of equipment/machines/props and so on.

- Target Muscle could be Either Upper Body's different Muscles or Lower Body's different Muscles or even Entire Body's Multiple Muscles, depending up on Many Factors again.

- Starting with Multi joint or Compound movements rather than single joint or concentration movements. Targeting Bigger Muscles first and step by step shifting towards Primary Supporting Muscles and if required Secondary supporting Muscles too, again this could be different for different people and always better to customise, depending on many factors and as per the demand or requirement or as per the situation.

- Apart from the Higher intensity levels, a greater number of sets and advance/superior exercises compared to Beginner Level's workout plan, other than these most of the points mentioned in the Beginner's level, may remain the same.

- And further progression in all the aspects like Muscle Strength, Muscle Endurance, Cardiovascular Endurance/ Stamina, Flexibility/ Mobility of Joints and Elasticity of Muscles/ Range of Motion, Reduced Recovery Period. With practice Muscles can achieve the ability to form less lactic acid or to wash out excess lactic acid by adapting different methods like Drinking Water during workouts, if the muscles get too contracted or pumped during workout doing some mild stretching, if required taking more rest in between 2 sets than usual, of Muscles and Speedy Recovery. And these things have to be the Target at all Fitness Levels.

And for those people who are actually Beginners, never worked out before I would like to suggest to start with Beginner Level only, no matter what your current fitness level is or what your age is or how great flexibility or shape of your body is. Never follow anyone's suggestions blindly if they suggest you to start with Intermediate or Advanced Workouts directly.

Also, for those, who have done the workouts in past on a regular basis and at advanced levels, but if there is a gap (No Activity or No Exercises at all) more than a Month, I would suggest them to start with beginner's level workouts for a while and then with progression they will be able to achieve the previous levels of fitness over the period of time. And if there is more gap, then I would recommend to start with conditioning and mobility routine first and then start with regular exercise routine as a beginner. Always remember that you have to start with simple and doable activities/exercises or as per the current body condition what is required. So that you will be able to maintain consistency. And once it becomes a habit it becomes sustainable workout for you and then you can easily progress in it with consistency.

But these are just the gross formats, cannot be considered as standards. There might be different sequence or odd combinations as per the requirement or wise choices as per the situation or as per the expertise and experience of the coach who designs the workout program. Safety and Effectiveness of the program completely depends on the wise and sensible thoughts of the Coach rather than just blindly followed science, also it depends up on client's consistency and response of the body to the program given and many more other factors.

Ideally one should start with a set of more number of repetition and low intensity or less weight/resistance and the exercise should target the bigger muscle or group of muscles and which require multi joint movement or compound movement and this set leads to sending the brain the signals that the targeted muscle or muscle group is at work and need support, so the brain gives more and more attention towards that particular area with every single attempt and supplies more blood flow which carries nutrition required and oxygen which helps in improved performance and faster recovery of that muscle or group of muscles. And with every set with increased load may lead to more attention, improved CNS function that means improved Mind Muscle coordination, increased blood circulation, more oxygen and improved function of the muscle with more strength and sustainability and improved performance and improved quality of movement.

That's why this flow or sequence is important - Warm up set, Preparatory set, Main Set and Final Set. And if one wants to target for higher weight or load in any particular exercise then he/she should add more preparatory sets with progressive overload if required.

And behind recommendation of these simple, suitable and sustainable exercises the main reason is your Safety.

If you start with very high intensity workouts or such exercises which don't match your current fitness levels, then it might be risky, it might be difficult for you to sustain for long term. If you start with Right kind of exercises, in the beginning itself using common sense, then your

further journey becomes much easy and sustainable. So always remember that, never go for higher numbers in the very first step itself, start with less, maintain it, achieve stability and then progress further.

Post Workout Stretches:

This is the most important part of any workout routine. But most of the time people underestimate it's great benefits. Many people just ignore it out of boredom or skip it because of lack of time or interest.

Let me tell you that this is the key factor for a great recovery.

Now people will wonder, how it can lead to a great recovery. Let me explain the reason and the very basic science behind it.

First of all, we will need to understand a simple mechanism, what happens exactly in a muscle while performing any set of exercise or while doing the movement where the muscle is in action and contracts to its maximal potential against resistance or overload. Basically, it is the tightening or shortening while contraction against resistance or in the concentric movement and lengthening or elongation of the muscle fibres against resistance at eccentric movement or at the controlled relaxing phase. This repetitive action in a set further leads to Maximal contraction, pump and tightness in the muscle, along with formation of 'Lactic Acid' as a biproduct in the muscle and it is a vital part or step of this entire process.

If more of lactic acid is formed in the muscle, the muscle becomes more fatigue, stiff, painful and more soared for that particular set or next few hours or even days depending up on the type and intensity of the workout as well as it also depends on an individual level and can take more time for recovery. But if a person does post workout stretches after an intense workout, then whatever lactic acid is formed and got accumulated into the muscles, get washed out towards lymph nodes and further for the excretion. If the muscle is stretched and elongated at its full capacity and maintained in that position on an average for at least 20 – 60 seconds or more, will help to wash out the lactic acid at maximum and let the fresh blood supply flow to the stretched muscles with more of Oxygen and More of Nutrition which always leads to a greater and faster recovery for sure.

Apart from this, post workout stretches improves the elasticity and makes your joints and muscles more flexible. And this improved flexibility leads to improved range of motion and target more area of muscles. And this leads to make the movement more effective.

Stretching helps to balance the muscles, helps to align the muscles and can also resolve issues occurred due to structural change in long run. And proper muscle balance helps to improve overall posture.

While stretching the focus automatically shifts on breathing and which helps to reduce stress on the muscles as well as on the mind, gradually.

Stretching actually reduces stress related pains or aches. Stretching leads to calm and peaceful feeling. Reduces Anxiety. Stretching Reduces risk of injuries. Stretching Reduces pain and muscle soreness. Post workout stretches leads to gradual cool down of the body.

Cooldown

Cooldown means, you need to actually cool your body down and bring back to the normal position as of before starting of the workouts.

For this you are supposed to lie down on the mat in calm and peaceful surroundings. Basically, it is called as 'Shavasan' in Yoga. If you have less time in hand you may do this for minimum 2 to 5 Minutes, but if you can spend more time on this you will be able to get the actual benefits of this. You may do an extended Shavasan for up to 20 Minutes. Actual technique to do Shavasan is as follows:

Step 1:

Body positioning/alignment

Place yourself in the most comfortable and relaxed position.

Feet apart, toes pointing outwards, as per your comfort.

Feet, hip joint, lower back, shoulders, neck and head placed in the most comfortable and relaxed position, so adjust your body parts and align yourself accordingly in the natural way.

Palms facing upwards, towards the ceiling.

Eyes Closed and Facial Muscles Relaxed.

Step 2:

Calm, Controlled and rhythmic Breathing.

After closing your eyes, focus on your breathing.

Feel your breathing.

Practice Deep Breathing (If Possible, otherwise do normal breathing in a controlled manner with more focus and Concentration).

Inhale…

Exhale Out….

Deep Inhale……

Deep Exhale Out with control.

Try to have a good control over your breathing.

And to gain more control over your breathing observe the gap in between inhalation and exhalation, every single time.

Practice, Slow, Steady, Rhythmic, Deep and Complete Breathing.

Feel Each and every single breath, which you inhale which you exhale out.

Every time you breath in feel the coolness of the inhaled fresh air. And every time you breath out feel the warmth of the exhaled air in the nostrils.

Follow and maintain the same pattern of breathing throughout.

Step 3:

Calm, Controlled and Positive Mental State.

Once you achieve the control over your breathing, continue breathing in the same right pattern throughout for the further progression in this meditative state.

Now shift your focus completely on your Mind.

First of all, calm down your mind and in this process, the right breathing pattern always helps.

Make your mind stable.

Now observe the current state of mind, you might observe that there are lots of random thoughts or one particular thought with depth or in detail or might be further complex state of thoughts.

If you don't practice any kind of meditation regularly and doing it for the first time, just observe the state of mind, as if you are sitting on a beach and observing the sea, observing the waves and tides which actually are your thoughts. And you might get engaged into the thought process by default. You might jump in to one of the tide or waves of the sea of thoughts and find yourself somewhere deep down in any of the thoughts. That's why always aim to sit back as an audience, try to get that control over your mind to not to get engaged in any of the thoughts and this you may achieve with regular practice. You just have to sit calm and observe the tides coming and going back. Observe the intensity of the Waves (thoughts) and how fast or slow they dissolve again.

If possible, stop the thought process, try to dissolve all the waves and tides and let the water be calm and clear like a lake or pond, so that you will be able to see the bottom. The bottom is filled with lot many things like your memories Good, Bad and Neutral. Spend some more time to have more calmness and clarity about your thoughts. Then Pick up the Good Memories and Positive thoughts, as if you are Picking up a Treasure

Box and Pearls from the bottom of the sea. Imagine positive situations which will lead towards a positive impact on your life. Try to explore beautiful and colourful species of fishes and other under water lives, beautiful flowers and plants.

With all these pleasurable and positive memories and thoughts, try to make yourself calmer and feel relaxed with your mind and with your entire body.

Step 4:

Fully Relaxed Body (In Extended Version of 'Shavasan' lasts long because there is more detailed relaxation method where there is more focus on relaxation of individual body parts).

Once you achieve the state of Calm and Controlled Mind, then shift the focus on the physical body. Start relaxing your entire body. Using the power of mind, command the body parts and starting from Lower body, feel and relax your legs. Then Feel and Relax your arms. Feel and Relax your Entire Back, right from Lower Back, Mid Back, Upper Back, Trapezius and Neck. Then Feel and Relax Abdomen Muscle and Side obliques, covering the entire stomach area. Then Feel and Relax Chest Muscles. Feel and relax both the shoulders, right and Left. Then feel and relax Neck and Throat. Then Feel and Relax, back of your head, top of the head and both the ears. And finally relax all your facial Muscles. Feel and relax your Forehead, feel and relax your eyebrows, feel and reax your eye lids and eye balls inside. Feel and relax your Nose and Nostrils. Feel and relax your lips. Feel and Relax your Chin and Cheeks. Now, you are feeling completely relaxed with all your facial muscles. Now just think about your overall entire body. Feel that your entire body is relaxed completely down.

Step 5:

Focus Shifting in Reverse order and be actually relaxed.

From Body to Mind and Mind to Breathing.

After relaxing each individual body part and overall full body. Shift your focus again on Mind, feel that Mind is calm, controlled and completely relaxed.

Then Shift the focus again from Mind to Breathing. Feel your breathing again, Inhale – Exhale Out. Deep inhale and compete exhale out with control, try to have a good control over your breathing again. Practice deep breathing again. Feel each and every single breath and try to make yourself completely relaxed with your mind and with your entire body. Just be with your own self. And maintain the same process for next 2 to 5 Minutes.

Step 6:

The Actual Relaxation -

Spend the actual time duration of 2 to 5 Minutes or 7 to 10 Minutes with your own-self. And follow the same process and make yourself completely relaxed with each and every single breath.

Step 7:

Step by Step, come back, out of the meditative state.

Now listen and follow the steps with full focus.

To come out of the Meditative Sleep State,

First of all, be aware of your breathing, Inhale and Exhale out. Feel your breathing again.

Then Shift your focus from breathing to Mind.

Be aware of Mind, recollect all your thoughts, restart your thought process, but start with positive thoughts, think about body and Mind's positive health and wellbeing.

Refresh your Mind.

Then Shift your focus from Mind to Body.

Be aware of your entire body, feel all your body parts which you have relaxed step by step. Right from your both the legs, both the Arms, Complete Spine and all the Muscles attached to your spine, Lower Back, Mid

Back, Upper back, trapezius, feel your Entire Back, then feel your Stomach, abdomen muscles, then feel your Chest and Shoulders, feel your Throat and Neck, then feel Back of your head, top of your head. And finally, feel all your facial muscles again one by one. Now just think about your overall entire body, feel your entire body. Observe all the body parts. Then do slight movements with your fingers and with your toes, feel your both the arms, feel your both the legs, feel your entire body.

Take your time and then very slowly turn to your Right side with your full body and stay in the same position for another 30 seconds. Then focus on your breathing again. Feel your breathing again, Deep Inhale, stay there watch the gap and count a couple of seconds and then Complete Exhale out with control and again after exhalation stay there watch the gap and count a couple of seconds and then complete inhale and repeat this practice. Practice deep breathing.

Note: Many people usually get confused or rather curious to know which side to turn after completion of Cooldown or Shavasan, Right side or Left Side and why to turn at Right Side? or why to turn at Left Side? So here is the answer to it. Our Right Nostril is the opening for or represents 'Surya Naadi'. Surya Naadi is responsible for Freshness, Activeness, alertness, aggression etc. so if in case you have done the workout in the morning and after this, you will be going to work then it is suggested to turn to 'Right Side'.

And to opposite of this, if you have done your workout in the evening or at night and after this you might not need to be much active or work or you are going to go to sleep after your dinner, then you should turn to left side and slowly get up, the reason behind it is that 'Left Nostril' opening represents 'Chandra Naadi' and it is responsible for calmness, slow and steady breath, relaxation and focus of mind as well as the body.

Step 8:

Getting Up

After 30 Seconds, take support of your hand and very slowly and gently come up and sit into Sukhasana or Vajrasana. Keep your eyes closed, with calm and controlled mind, controlled breathing. Maintain the same position for at least 20 seconds and then start with 'Omkar' or Chanting 'Om', in case if you have no time to do Pranayama.

Pranayama:

After you got up from 'Shavasana' and Sitting in any 'Aadharasana' like 'Sukhasan' or 'Vajrasan'. You may start with some basic Pranayama (Breathing Exercises) with low intensity and as per your comfort and Limitations.

You may do few basic variations like:

Kapaal Bhaati: Forcefully Exhalation with intense strokes through nose only. Simultaneously subconscious inhalation should happen automatically. And at the same time your stomach will be sucked or pulled inside with each stroke automatically or by default.

Those with, medical condition like Asthma, Hypertension (High Blood Pressure) and Complications related with breathing and Lungs, should avoid it completely or do it with very mild strokes and 1 stroke per second or per breath but make sure that the intensity of the stroke while exhalation should be very low and comfortable. Still if feel uncomfortable, then stop.

Repetitions: If you can do it properly and with good speed then 100 to 300 should be the target.

For beginners: You may start with low or moderate intensity and 2 to 3 or up to 5 or 10 stokes per breath as per your capacity, you need to be wise enough to understand what is your limit, what is safe for you. You may do, 50 to 150 times.

Anulom Vilom: Anulom Vilom is basically balancing, Surya Naadi and Chandra Naadi. **Anulom Vilom** is a specific type of pranayama, or controlled breathing formula, in yoga. It involves holding one nostril closed while inhaling from the other and then holding the other nostril closed while exhaling from the first one. The ideal, correct, easy and the most basic way of doing Anulom Vilom is:

Aadharasana (Basic sitting pose) - Vajrasan/ Sukhasan/ Ardha-padmasana/ Padmasana (In case if you are not able to sit in any of these Aadharasana then just sit into a chair or sit on a bed normally, but make sure that you are supposed to sit straight keeping your spine erect and neck into neutral position and facial muscles and other body parts in relaxed position. Then using your right thumb close your right nostril, then inhale from left nostril using the full capacity of your lungs, once you inhale completely and filled the lung full of air then hold there observe the gap for a couple of seconds, then open the right nostril and immediately close the left nostril with the ring finger and small finger of the same right hand and complete exhale out and empty the lungs completely from the open side, the right nostril, then be there and hold the breath out only for a couple of seconds, observe the gap, then inhale with the same nostril right one with fullest capacity, fill the lungs and hold the breath for a couple of seconds observe the gap and close the right nostril with right thumb and open the left nostril immediately and exhale out with full capacity from left side and hold the breath out for couple of seconds and observe the gap. This makes one complete round of Anulom Vilom. As per your capacity and will you may do 1 round or repeat up to 5 or 7 rounds and consider it as a set. You may repeat up to 3 such sets.

Bhramari: Bhramari is basically a Vibrational Frequency created by using a unique method, we may also consider it as a kind of sound vibration therapy to improve the functions of brain, activate or stimulate most of the parts of brain by the vibrations created, these vibrations sensitise the nerves and makes them stronger and improves their functions inside the area of forehead and overall brain. Increases concentration and focus. By regular practice of Bhramari, you can get rid of Insomnia, headaches, Stress, depression, anxiety and get the benefits of improved sleep, improved memory and improved concentration etc.

Now let's see, how can we do Bhramari in the easiest and correct way:

Aadharasana (Basic sitting pose) – Vajrasan/ Sukhasan/ Ardha-padmasana/ Padmasana (In case if you are not able to sit in any of these Aadharasana then just sit into a chair or sit on a bed normally, but make sure that you are supposed to sit straight keeping your spine erect and neck into neutral position and facial muscles and other body parts in relaxed position. Close your eyes, then using your thumbs close the openings of both the ears, either by putting the thumbs inside the ear holes gently and keep a very gentle pressure applied throughout, but make sure that the ears shouldn't get hurt due to grown nails, nails should be trimmed properly, don't apply too much pressure, just see that you should not be able to hear any noise around you. Or the other way to just press the thumbs around the openings of ears and try to close it, again, don't apply too much pressure. Then keep your both hands' index fingers lose and with other 3 fingers of right and left hands on the right and left eyes respectively and try to cover the closed eyes with a very gentle pressure, do not press very hard or tight. Make sure the elbows are lifted alongside the body stretched backwards opening up the ribcage and keeping the elbows aligned with the shoulders. Maintain the same pose throughout the set. Now keeping the mouth shut, lips closed and touching each other means, without opening the mouth, try to chant 'Om' in an extended form, so that because of closed lips it will sound like "Hmmmmm......!" and will create very good vibrations all over inside the mouth, throat area, head and brain as well. After completion of the sound made once, be in the same position, don't remove hands or change the position, just inhale completely and slowly with exhalation again create the sound of 'Om' and try to extend it as much as possible in one breath but as per your capacity and limit. And repeat the same process again. You may do a set or 3 or 5 or 7 or up to 11 depending upon an individual choice, will and comfort. Once done with a set remove hands, relax, breathe slowly and calmly. Take rest for at least 30 to 60 seconds and then you may go for another set, you may do 2-3 sets.

Chanting 'Om' / 'Omkar':

After having a Focused Mind and controlled breathing, deep inhale and start with chanting 'Om'.

One 'Om' per breath.

For each and every single chanting, try to sound loud and clear, try to extend as much as possible, but within your limit and capacity. Feel the vibrations every single time.

Do 3 times or 5 times or 7 or 11 or even 21 times as you feel comfortable.

After completion of the desired number of chanting 'Om', Keep your eyes closed, feel the vibrations created by this sound, focus again on your breathing, feel your breathing again, inhale and exhale out, maintain the same process for another 20 Seconds.

After 20 seconds, keep your eyes still closed, then rub your palms on each other vigorously and try to generate heat on the rubbing portions. Then place your heated palms on your eyes and on overall your face, feel the heat of the palms and then slowly open your eyes.

Finally Done with your entire workout including everything, covering all aspects of Fitness.

Wise sequence of workouts

Now let me tell you the Ideal sequence, as per my Understanding and Experience. If you have many options to choose from, then choose the safest and most effective options wisely and sensibly:

1st Stage of the Warm up:

- Always start with the 'Basic Joint Mobility Drills' covering all major joints and muscle groups right from 'Head to Toe'. And this has to be done in a slow, steady and in a rhythmic and Controlled manner, if the sequence is followed ideally from Neck Joint to Ankle joint it will be Beneficial. Especially when you are doing the workout in the Morning Time after a Good sleep and Rest of 6-8 Hrs or Even if you are doing the workouts in the Evening Time after an 8 Hrs of Stressful Office work.

- If you are going to do Weight Training as your main workout in the Morning Time, then you should spend more time for Warm up, because the body is completely relaxed after the sleep. So, it requires more preparation, especially if the intensity of the weight training is more or high.

The ideal workouts for the Morning Time after 6 to 8 Hrs' sleep should be Basically, Yoga and Pranayam or Moderate intensity or Brisk Walking or a Combination of both Walking followed by Yoga and Pranayam and Meditation. This has to be done outdoor and in an open and airy area where there would be a direct exposure to the Sun and Fresh Air, the best examples of such places are as follows, A Garden, surrounded by a lot of trees, A beach with Fresh air and Exposure to Sun, A Hill Side area or any suitable outdoor area, where there is direct exposure to sun and fresh air. And one should must add a Cooldown/Shavasana for short time to make the body back to Normal conditions in terms of Heart rate, Breathing, Blood Circulation and Body temperature, ideally one should bring back all the things mentioned above to Normal, before Starting Yoga, if you have completed the cardio or any other workouts.

So, the ideal time for Yoga is Morning.

And the ideal time for weight training is in the evening. Because, if you are in the flow of movements (Includes Macro as well as Micro Movements) throughout the day time, and by the time of evening body can be in a good condition in terms of blood circulation, mobility of different joints and muscles, so it requires less time and less efforts to warm up and prepare the body for the workouts especially for the Weight Training compared to Morning time, provided if you spend Minimum time in A/C (Air conditioning – Cool Temperature, which may make the muscles and joints stiff).

So, we can say Evening is the more Ideal Time for Weight Training.

- Then Followed by Moderate Intensity Cardio (Brisk Walk, Running or any Cardio Machine or Indoor Cardio Activities like Jumping Jack/Skipping/Sport Marching depending up on the Fitness levels, on an individual basis etc) And the Time duration may range in between 5 Minutes to 10 Minutes.

- **2nd stage of warm up**:

Body flow like Surya Namaskar or a Body Flow Power Yoga Circuit or World's Greatest stretch or any other specific stretches or drills or Dynamic Stretching or any particular movement or exercise like free squats or push-ups or combination of both (Burpees) or Hindu Push-ups (Dand/ Dive bombs) etc. Depending up on the intensity of the workouts or the Target Muscle or Group of Muscles. Or depending upon multiple other aspects and freedom of choice.

OR

In the 2nd Stage, you may also do Core Strengthening Exercises along with few Floor exercises targeting the Abdomen, Side Obliques and Lower Back Muscles along with some standard Exercises like Forearm Planks, Side Planks, Boat Pose and Glute Bridge depending up on the fitness level or body limitations, there might be alterations in the type of exercises and intensity levels.

OR

And those with any injuries or postural defect, structural or muscle imbalance, can work on the specific workouts or exercises or stretches or mobility drills which will help them in healing, recovery or balancing the muscles or structural alignment by regular practice. And due to this kind of body limitations or stiffness are not able to perform the normal way of 2nd stage of warm up or even beginners also should avoid it in the very beginning phase, once they start with their workout routine.

Some people might choose the 1st option or some might like to do the second option and some might be interested in doing both. Again, it depends on the choice of the person and Fitness levels or body limitations or Time available in hand.

1st Stage of Main Workout:

In this stage, basically one should do Preparation for the main sets (either 1 or 2 Number of sets). As mentioned earlier in the previous chapter, Whether the person is going to do a full body workout at beginner level or intermediate or if it's targeting Upper Body or Lower Body or any specific Muscle or muscle group, one should always start with the biggest muscle, until and unless there is any strategy or a thought is involved to start in a different way, then in that case there is a complete freedom of selection of exercises or starting with any specific muscle or group of muscles.

These preparatory sets could be 1 or 2 or 3 also with gradual but slight increment in the weight or intensity in every set and slight decrease in number of reps in every set of that particular exercise, depending up on the intensity of the Final Set. If the person is really going to do the Final set very heavy then he/she needs a greater number of sets for preparation and this might be different for different people.

2nd stage of Main Workout:

This is actually the beginning of main workout and at this stage, after completion of preparatory sets of the very first exercise we are supposed to do **Main Sets**, some people might do just 1 main set and some might do **Main Set 1** and **Main Set 2** as well, (again depending upon the intensity of the Final Set) of this particular exercise. And in this stage the Poundage/Weight/Intensity increases further more compared to the preparatory sets and it's quite challenging, with reduced rep range. Number of rep range and choice of weight is completely depending up on the fitness level of the person and few other factors.

3rd Stage of Main Workout:

At this stage of Main Workout, you are supposed to do the Final Set, utilising fullest capacity and with maximum Poundage/Weight/Intensity and obviously the repetition range would be minimal/lowest by default. And this Final set is just One and last for the first exercise.

And for all the further exercises which are mentioned by your Coach/Trainer are supposed to do only 2 to 3 Sets each with Gradual increment in weights/Poundage/Intensity and reduction in the repetition range. Covering-up and targeting the major muscles, then followed by supporting muscles, then secondary supporting muscles in the descending order 2 to 3 sets of each exercise targeting these muscles till the end of the main workout. (In some cases, people do more, lets say 4-6 number of sets of the one particular exercise rather than doing a variety of exercises and in that case they do very few variations but with a greater number of sets to complete focus and to target deep muscles.)

1st Stage of Cooldown:

As per different thoughts and availability of time and depending on multiple factors, people may break this stage into 2 parts Cooldown Option A and B. Let's see in details.

Cooldown, Option A:

Some people may prefer to do a Moderate intensity cardio and the ideal time duration is from 5 Minutes to 20 Minutes, depending up on multiple factors, but most important factors are, a) Availability of time, b) Intensity of the main workout done as well as the intensity of the cardio workout to be done for cooldown and c) Fitness goal.

End of the day its completely depending upon the choice of the person.

Let me clear this point also, many people have a misconception about post workout cardio. Some people think that Post workout Cardio helps in Fat Burn/Calorie Burn, some people think that doing post workout cardio can result in Muscle loss. Both the things mentioned could be possible at some extent and the ratio of this possibility is very less, until and unless the person is doing it in excess and at an extreme level, then it might be risky beyond the mentioned time duration and intensity levels. If we talk about Muscle loss in specific, then that completely depends up on the body type and diet (Protein-Carbs ratio) and other important factors.

The main reason, why I mentioned this point and recommend to do Moderate intensity Cardio in the limited time duration is that, it will help to remove Lactic acid from the muscles, which by default accelerate the recovery process.

It completely depends upon personal choice to do post workout or directly go for the post workout stretches (Cooldown – Option – B) after the completion of Main Workout.

Cooldown, Option B:

In this stage, we are supposed to do Post Workout Stretches to Relax the Muscles, to increase the elasticity/flexibility of the target Muscle or group of muscles. And it also contributes to improve on the range of motion or mobility of a particular joint/joints which are related to the target muscle/group of muscles.

We can categorise the stretches into 2 parts:

A) **Active Stretches**: Stretches done by self, as per the requirement of the main workout done & targeted muscles.

B) **Passive Stretches:** Stretches (technically correct and by understanding the limitations, stiffness of the person and in 'Pain free' range, from the safety point of view) given by another person (Coach/Trainer/Workout Buddy), as per the Main workout done.

Post Workouts Stretches helps in removal of lactic acid from the muscles and bring in the fresh blood supply to the stretched muscles/group of muscles, which by default accelerates the speed of recovery.

2nd Stage of Cooldown:

After completion of Post Workout Stretches, we are supposed to do Stretches for the Core Muscle Group, irrespective of the workout done in the main workout and followed by the post workout stretches targeting those muscles used. And we are supposed to do these stretches for core muscles group on every workout day. Focus on proper stretches of Core Muscles Group which includes Hip Muscles' Group, Groin Muscles, Abdomen Muscle, Side Oblique Muscles and Lower Back Muscles etc., in order to attain a greater conditioning of core group and maintain it by regular practice.

3rd Stage of Cooldown:

Shavasana/ Subconscious Sleep:

This stage of Cooldown is very important, where we cover Shavasana/ Subconscious Sleep. Time duration from Minimum 5 Minutes to 20 Minutes (Depending upon the availability of time). In this stage we achieve the Normal Pace of Breathing, Heart Beats and also Neutralise the blood flow and equal blood circulation towards all body parts equally covering upper extremity and lower extremity. This stage actually helps in reducing fatigue, soreness, tiredness and makes one refreshed with Mind and the entire body and stores energy. For detailed information or reference please check the previous chapter.

1st Stage of Revitalisation (Initiation for the recovery process):

Breathing Exercises / Pranayam:

Stick to basic breathing exercises which are simple/easy to do and with moderate intensity. Follow the instructions and process correctly. Some best examples of easy breathing exercises are as follows:

A) **Kapaal Bhaati**

B) **Anulom Vilom**

C) **Bhramari**

All the 3 breathing techniques explained in details in the previous chapter, please check for reference and more information about the same.

Do Pranayam as per your comfort and ease. Never push yourself too hard or never try to do it at an extreme level, in terms of intensity or number of repetitions or number of sets. As an important part of a complete workout, limit the intensity, time duration and repetitions. Always focus on the quality rather than quantity.

In this stage the supply of oxygen increases after an exhausting main workout. It actually makes you feel refreshed and recharged. And this practice also, makes you feel Fresh and Energetic again.

2nd Stage of Revitalisation:

Chanting 'OM' / Omkar:

Chanting 'Omkar' helps you to refresh, as well as tune yourself with the right vibes/ frequency of the universe that provides you with the positive energy, clarity of thoughts, a calm, controlled mind and a great aura around you.

After the 'Omkar', you may continue with a short duration Meditation catching the last vibrations felt while chanting the 'Om' and continue with it by focusing more on these vibrations and go into the meditative phase.

3rd Stage of Revitalisation:

Meditation:

Continuing from the same state, stage and pose from chanting 'Om', you should start with the meditation.

Meditation is a practice that can help you relax, focus, and cultivate a sense of inner peace. Here is a step-by-step guidance for a short meditation session that you carry out up to 10 Minutes:

1. Sit with straight spine but relaxed body position. Keep your eyes closed and soften your gaze inside the eye lids.

2. Continue the flow of deep breaths, inhaling through your nose and exhaling through your nose only. With each exhale, release any tension in your body and allow yourself to sink deeper into relaxation. So, focus more on the exhalation part.

3. Bring your attention to your breath. Notice the sensation of the air moving in and out of your nostrils or the rise and fall of your belly or focus on your heart beats and feel them. You can count your breaths, starting with one on the inhale and two on the exhale, up to ten, and then

start again. Watch the gap in between one inhalation and one exhalation this will help you to focus more on your breath, have a great control over it and which will lead to calm your mind down.

4. Your mind may wander, and that's okay. When you notice that your thoughts have drifted away from your breath, gently bring your attention back to your breath without judgment.

5. To increase the effectiveness and focus, just observe the gap in between your breathes again. Count the seconds during the gap in between 1 inhalation and 1 exhalation. This the most effective technique to increase the focus, concentration, to calm the mind down and to keep any thoughts away from intervention.

6. Continue to meditate for as long as you feel comfortable. If you're new to meditation, start with just a few minutes, and gradually increase the duration as you get more comfortable with the practice.

7. When you're ready to end your meditation, take a few deep breaths, stretch your body, then rub your palms for few seconds make some heat created due to rubbing and the palms become warm, then place these warm palms on your closed eyes wait for few more seconds then

move your palms on all over your face neck, shoulders, arms, chest, try to cover the area of back as well, thighs and feet too, but without changing your position, once you move your palms from all over the body and then slowly open your eyes.

Meditation is a practice, and it takes time and consistency to develop. Don't worry if you find it difficult at first, keep practicing, and be patient with yourself.

4ᵗʰ Stage of Revitalisation:

Sing or Say a Prayer:

1. Once you are done with the meditation, you have almost made a connection with your own inner self or at soul level and now it's time to get connected with nature or universe or with the God. Say or sing a prayer if you know any. But here is the twist, do not pray for your own self. Pray for someone else or others or for the entire world and universe in general. In any form. In any language. Your prayer will be herd for sure and it will come true.

2. Once you are done with your prayer, just be grateful or Thank to the God or Universe or the Nature for no reason and for every possible reason.

And this is the last and final stage of your workout which you have done to be 'Quantum Fit'.

This means that you have covered all the aspects to achieve Fitness of your Physical Body, Mental Body, Emotional Body, Spiritual Body and Etheric Body.

This is the way to attain a great balance and be neutral with all forms and all bodies we have got, to become **'Quantum Fit'.**

Ideal workout suggestions as per Ayurvedic wisdom considering 'Tridoshas'

As per the Ayurvedic knowledge and wisdom, the human body is seen as a microcosm of the larger universe, and it is believed that the same fundamental principles that govern the natural world also govern the human body. One of the key principles in Ayurveda is the concept of doshas, which are three fundamental energies that govern all physiological and psychological functions in the body. The three doshas are Vata, Pitta, and Kapha.

Temperature and weather conditions as per the location or season, can have a significant impact on the doshas in the body. For example, extreme cold temperatures can increase Vata dosha, while hot temperatures can increase Pitta dosha. Cold temperatures can also cause Kapha dosha to accumulate in the body, while hot temperatures can increase and aggravate Pitta dosha. When the doshas are imbalanced due to weather or temperature, it can cause various health issues. For example, an imbalance in Vata dosha can lead to constipation, dry skin and anxiety, while an imbalance in Pitta dosha can cause irritability, inflammation, and fever. An imbalance in Kapha dosha can cause lethargy, weight gain and congestion. In Ayurveda, it is important to maintain a great balance of the doshas by adapting to different weather conditions and temperature changes. This can be achieved through various measures such as eating a balanced diet, practicing meditation, some easy physical exercises and yoga, and using specific fruits, vegetables, herbs and oils that help to balance the doshas.

Exercise is an essential component of a health and lifestyle, and the type of exercise that is best for an individual depends on their body type and dosha imbalances. It also depends on the type of climate, whether hot or cold or seasonal temperature. The weather, temperature, and climate can also affect the ideal workouts for an individual. Here are some suggestions for ideal workouts or exercises based on different weather conditions and dosha types:

1. **Extreme Heat:**

    - Individuals with a **dominant Pitta dosha should avoid intense or high-impact workouts like HIIT, during extreme heat** as it can further increase Pitta and lead to dehydration. Instead, they should **opt for more gentle exercises such as swimming, walking, or yoga.**

- For individuals with a **dominant Kapha dosha, high-intensity exercises such as HIIT, Weight Training, interval training or kickboxing can be beneficial** as it helps to boost metabolism and improve energy levels.
- Individuals with a **dominant Vata dosha should avoid exercising during the hottest part of the day** and instead **opt for more grounding exercises such as Tai Chi, Pilates, Slow pace Suryanamaskars, Power Yoga or simple yoga asanas etc.**

2. **Extreme Cold:**

- Individuals with a **dominant Vata dosha should focus on exercises that are warming and grounding, such as Indoor cycling, yoga, Power Yoga, Suryanamaskars etc.** They should also dress in warm layers to avoid aggravating Vata dosha.
- For individuals with a **dominant Kapha dosha, high-intensity exercises such as Aerobics, cardio or HIIT workouts, weight training, circuit training etc,** can be beneficial as it helps to increase metabolism and reduce lethargy.

- Individuals with a **dominant Pitta dosha should opt for exercises that are not too intense, such as Yoga, walking, indoor weightlifting using light weights (with proper rest in between sets) etc**, to avoid further increasing Pitta dosha.

3. **Moderate Temperatures:**

   - Individuals with a **dominant Vata dosha should focus on exercises that are grounding and gentle, such as yoga or light/low intensity weightlifting.**
   - For individuals with a **dominant Kapha dosha, a combination of strength training and cardio exercises can be beneficial to maintain a healthy weight and metabolism.**
   - Individuals with a **dominant Pitta dosha should opt for exercises that are not too intense and that focus on balance and flexibility, such as yoga or Pilates.**

It is important for individuals to listen to their bodies and adjust their workouts accordingly, based on how they feel. It is also recommended to consult with a qualified Ayurvedic practitioner along with an experienced fitness expert (who is wise and has a belief in ancient science, techniques of natural healing and has a great understanding and knowledge about human body at quantum levels), to determine the ideal workouts based on their unique body type and dosha imbalances.

Also know that each dosha has its own time of day when it is dominant and active in the body. The following is a breakdown of the ideal times for various activities based on the dosha dominance:

1. **Vata Dosha:**

    - Vata is dominant from 2 am to 6 am and from 2 pm to 6 pm.
    - The morning Vata period (2 am to 6 am) is the ideal time for Pranayam, meditation, introspection, and creative pursuits.
    - The afternoon Vata period (2 pm to 6 pm) is a good time for physical activity such as yoga or walking. Recommended light and grounding exercises like yoga, pilates, slow pace Suryanamaskars, free hand exercises or floor exercises from low to moderate intensity etc.

2. **Pitta Dosha:**

    - Pitta is dominant from 10 am to 2 pm and from 10 pm to 2 am.

- The midday Pitta period (10 am to 2 pm) is the ideal time for mental work, decision making, and problem solving, one can actually do Meditation during this time, it would be more effective and beneficial.
- The night time Pitta period (10 pm to 2 am) is the ideal time for sleep and relaxation, meditation also can be done and Subconscious relaxation can be done in the form of 'Yog Nidra' or 'Subconscious Sleep'.

3. **Kapha Dosha:**

- Kapha is dominant from 6 am to 10 am and from 6 pm to 10 pm.
- The morning Kapha period (6 am to 10 am) is a good time for exercise and physical activity to help stimulate the body. Weight Training, Cardio and other forms of exercises can be done.
- The evening Kapha period (6 pm to 10 pm) is a good time for winding down, relaxation, and preparing for sleep. Meditation can be done and Subconscious relaxation can be done in the form of 'Yog Nidra' or 'Subconscious Sleep' also can be done.

These timings suggested are in general and these guidelines may vary depending upon individual factors such as age, lifestyle, and health. If an individual has a dosha imbalance, these guidelines may not apply as they may need to focus on balancing the affected dosha.

Following a daily routine that aligns with the dominant dosha at each time of day can help to maintain balance in the body and promote overall health and well-being.

Wise understanding about the 'Process of Results'

Process of Result in simple language is 'Work in Progress'. And this means you still have to continue working on your fitness journey to achieve your health and fitness goals, regardless of results (Positive or Negative). And never ever be confused about it. Even if you are still stuck to the same weight, in spite of regular exercising and dieting since last 6 Month, never ever think to quit, if you are doing the workouts regularly from last 6 Months, that means you have progressed in terms of mental strength, determination and progressed in putting efforts to maintain the required consistency with great amount of discipline. This means you are on the 'Right Track', and achieved success in few aspects required.

Let me explain you about the wise idea of the Result or Progression:

Don't think that weight is the only criteria to gauge your progress or results, it is just a tiny parameter amongst many other important parameters.

You should know exact and important ways of tracking your Progress. And this will help you to change your mind set and approach towards your Fitness Journey, very positively. You perception is important.

Here is a Lesson for you all, which will be helpful for lifetime. The very first important thing is to understand, what to expect from the efforts you put throughout your fitness journey. Know exactly what are the benefits apart from just weight loss or inch loss.

Find out the reason for which you have started your fitness journey.

And this will be the greatest motivation for you to continue your fitness journey irrespective of the results.

Let me explain, how the tracking of results or progress help us:

Results or progress is just to know where we stand, that means whether we are on Right Path or Not. Good Results Motivate us and generally bad results may demotivate us, but still, we have to continue our fitness journey with patience and dedication.

Tracking the results (Positive or Negative) helps to decide what should be your next strategy. We come to know, where do we stand. This is how you are able to Gauge your Current Fitness Levels.

Progress:

Progress can be called, as a Positive Change in internal Systems which are responsible for condition of health and overall body, right from the cell level everywhere internally, superficial view or visibility of the body, psychology or the mind set or approach towards health and fitness And the improved connection with your own self as well as with your surroundings and this is achieved or can be achieved by constant practice of Right kind of combination exercises which are customized and are made most suitable for you as per your current fitness levels, physical appearance and body symmetry, considering your strengths, limitations and the ability to adapt these set of exercises over a certain period of time and which always leaves a scope, for further improvements. Most important aspect here which we need understand with a broad vision is that, Progress cannot be measured or counted in a certain range of Numbers, because we are dealing with the most complex design in the whole universe, in fact the whole universe is placed inside this Unique Machine called 'The Human Body', with constant changes at every fraction of seconds and at the cell levels, so it's very difficult to give accuracy or even approximated 'Values or Numbers'. But the Progress can be definitely felt internally and be seen superficially.

Understand the criteria of result/ progress:

- Body Weight on the Scale
- Body Measurements
- Body Mass Index (BMI – Fat % and Muscle Mass ratio)
- Fitness Test (Includes: Muscle Strength Test – Upper Body and Lower Body, Muscle Endurance Test – Core Muscles, Cardiovascular Endurance Test and Flexibility Test etc.)
- In case of any Medical Conditions or Lifestyle Disorders (Like Hypertension, Diabetes, Thyroid Condition, Cholesterol, PCOD/PCOS, Respiratory Disorders etc and so on), Reversal of it and Regularised or Normal/Improved Functioning of Internal systems and which can be gauged by some of the following Reports/Tests e.g., Thyroid, Sugar, Liver Functioning, Cholesterol, Blood Pressure etc and so on…
- In Case of Surgeries or Physical Injuries or Physical Limitations or Postural Defect (By Birth or By Improper Workstyle, Poor postures and Muscle loss due to lack of exercise and muscle imbalance): After Sensible Customization of planned workout schedule, Gaining Strength, Mobility, Flexibility, Conditioning, Improved Postures, Core

Strength and Proper Functioning of the affected Muscle or joint or Body parts. E.g. – Recovery in Knee Injury, Shoulder Injuries, Hip Joint Injuries, Spondylitis, Knee Caving/Knocked Knees, Hernia etc and so on.

The common and superficial understanding of results for commoners:

- Weight
- Belly Fat or Fat reduction from any specific area.
- 6 Packs Abs or Flat Stomach
- Shredded Body
- Increased Muscles
- Big Biceps
- Toning and Tightness in the body
- Lean Muscles, lean body
- Athletic body

Common expectations from common people:

- Super-fast Results
- Gain Super Powers immediately
- Fast weight loss
- Fast weight gain
- Start with very advanced workouts or Functional training Or CrossFit or at the same

level where you had reach once when you were consistency and had achieved advance level by putting efforts for a couple of years.

- Feeling of, half of the work is done just by doing the payments for any fitness program or gym membership and want to see instant results without taking any efforts or without spending sufficient required time or without going through necessary process in order to achieve the fitness goal.

Common Mistakes which affect results:

- Focus only on 1 or 2 aspects of Fitness and ignoring all of the other.
- Being too choosy.
- Being too lazy.
- Not having a serious approach.
- Doing the exercises just for fun and entertainment.
- Not listening to the experts.
- Not trusting the experts or the process or the plan.
- By being always confused.
- Never getting satisfied by even achieving good results.
- Underestimate own selves and the experts.

- Being too greedy for results.
- **Over Training:** Anything excess leads to some sort of problem, that's why try to balance things.
- **People do underestimate:**

    a) **Warmup:** Basic cardio activity and joint mobility drills, micro movements, to prepare the body for the main workouts by increasing the heart rate up-to necessary levels, increase blood circulation in target area, increase the viscosity of synovial fluid in the joints etc.

    b) **Strengthening and conditioning:** Strengthening and conditioning of minor muscles, internal/deep muscles, supporting muscles or group of muscles, ligaments, joints and core muscles' group, which includes lower back muscles, abdomen muscles and some part of the hip/glute muscles' group. Also strengthening and conditioning of every single movable joint present in the body is very important in all age groups especially in adults and senior citizens.

    c) **Post workout stretching:** Improves flexibility and removes lactic acid (most common bi product forms in the muscles during exercise).

d) **Proper cooldown:** Very important to neutralise and regularise the blood circulation, normalises breathing, normalises heartbeat, reduce physical stress and reduces mental stress.

There could be difference in results considering the following list of factors:

- Age
- Gender
- Body type
- Bone density
- Body weight
- Height (In case of growing children)
- Goal specific or goal-oriented exercise program
- Medical condition
- Physical limitations
- Injuries
- Mental blocks or psychology
- Emotional Blocks and psychology affecting motivational levels
- Stress levels (physical stress or psychological stress), etc.

Actual Parameters to gauge or track one's progression:

- Difference in weight (weight loss or weight gain as per the fitness goal).
- Muscle gain/ muscle building.
- Inch loss/ difference in measurements.
- Strengthening of internal or small muscles or group of muscles.
- Conditioning of important supporting muscles and ligaments and joints.
- Flexibility and mobility of group of muscles and joints.
- Improved reflexes/ improved mind muscle coordination.
- Improved functioning of CNS (central nervous system).
- Improved core muscles' group strength and functional strength.
- Better/ improved balance.
- Improved internal systems (respiratory, cardio vascular, blood Circulation, digestive, reproductive, etc.).
- Improved metabolism of almost every system and almost all hormones.
- Hormonal balance.

- Improved absorption of nutrients.
- Improved oxygen intake, supply and absorption at all levels.
- Immunity at its best.
- Building of new cells.
- Muscles' building.
- Increased basal metabolic rate (BMR).
- Fat % drop down.
- Lymphic system at its best functions.
- Decreased visceral fat.
- In many cases, regular exercising could be a reversal for lifestyle disorders like hypertension, diabetes, thyroid, PCOD (Poly Cystic Ovarian Disease) or PCOS (Poly Cystic Ovarian Syndrome).
- Increased appetite.
- Improved quality of sleep.
- Reduced recovery period.
- Fast recovery from physical injuries (by customized rehab exercise routine)
- Fast recovery from wounds.
- Can achieve Acid-alkali balance, with regular exercises (Combination of strength exercises, cardio, yoga, pranayama etc) along with a balanced diet.

- Improved Posture.
- Structural alignment.
- Balanced muscles (especially opposite muscles – agonist and antagonist muscles).
- Improved confidence.
- Achieve great physique.
- Improved personality features or characteristics.

Accelerate or boost up the process of results:

- **Starting right:** By starting with right kind of workouts and with a sensible approach, which is customised and most suitable as per your fitness goal and current fitness levels and designed as per the situation, considering physical limitations or medical conditions (if any).
- **Maintaining the consistency:** Know that, consistency is the key factor and plays an important role in the process of result and progress.
- **Avoid Overdoing:** By not overdoing anything, by limiting the workouts and not doing too much or trying too many things at a stretch or all at once. And this simple factor helps you to get the most important benefits of 'Endorphins', the feelgood hormones.

- **Step by step Progression:** Do what is necessary as per the time and situation. Live in the present moment first and then think of the next step to improvise or progress.

- **No Showing Off:** Do the workouts for the sake of your own self and not for anybody else. Never do your workouts for showing off or just to satisfy your ego. Be matured enough to understand this very simple fact that, your body is your own and nobody else owns it, so you are the owner of this property (body). So, have a common sense to understand about the things which are beneficial and are into your capacity or limit and the things which may create damage or be harmful to your body. So be matured, be wise to be 'Quantum Fit'.

- **Listen to your body and mind:** Always try to understand and observe your own body. Understand the signals given by your body and wisely understands your own feelings. Address your own gut feelings. And act accordingly or take wise decision.

- **No Comparison:** Do not compare yourself with anybody.

- **No Competition:** Do not compete with anyone else risking your body and health or even life.

- **Open your eyes:** Do not blindly follow any trend or anyone, if it's not safe for you and not suitable to you as per your current fitness level, situation or by considering many other factors. Be wise, open your eyes and see what is right and what is wrong for your own fitness, health and wellness.
- **Safety in Simplicity:** Believe in simple and sustainable workouts, don't fall for risky and complicated variations.
- Improve mind, muscle coordination.
- **Right Techniques keep you safe always:** Improve on techniques and never just keep overloading every time, beyond your capacity.
- **Repair before further rupture:** Let the full recovery happen from the soreness or last workout done and then only continue with your next progressive workout session. Always give sufficient required time and rest for recovery from the damage.
- **BREAK THE PLATEAU:** Learn and implement different techniques to break the plateau in your workout routine.
- **MAKE SENSIBLE AND REQUIRED, RIGHT KIND OF CHANGES IN YOUR WORKOUTS OVER THE PERIOD OF**

TIME: Learn and implement the techniques of **'PERIODIZATION'**.

- **Attend Natural Calls:** Eat when you feel hungry, drink water or liquids and fluids when you feel thirsty, sleep when you feel sleepy. Try to attend all-natural calls, in terms of hunger, thirst and sleep, whenever possible for you. Follow these simple things and see a great change in your fitness and health in long run.

- Stay Natural always.

- **Too Calculative = Too Stressful:** Don't overthink about the result or it's process. Don't be very calculative, about calories (Consumed or Burnt), about body weight, measurement and so on.

- **Do not expect too much:** Accept the reality about the situation, with a positive approach.

- **Petrochemical Based Medicines come with side effects:** Don't fall for unnecessarily medications consisting petrochemical base. Never Ever take **steroids** or other harmful medications. Think about your own future, think long term side effects. Think about your family. **DO NOT RISK YOUR LIFE, FITNESS and HEALTH**, for the sake of temporary benefits.

- **Being simple is simply effective:** Think every aspect of your fitness journey and keep it simple and sustainable yet effective.
- **Value for Health and Wealth:** Hiring a right guide, in your fitness journey will lead you to reach your destination in less time with safety and make your journey enjoyable and memorable. Hiring a Fitness Expert or coach or an experienced personal trainer is very important and valuable step in achieving your fitness goals and make your fitness journey successful. If you can afford, you can always pay a good amount of fees to reward your fitness expert or coach for his/her efforts based on their knowledge, experience, wisdom and professionalism. And enjoy the most fruitful benefits and have a great balance of a great level of fitness, health and wellness at quantum level.

  If you can afford to have a lavish dinner in a luxury hotel or throw a party every now and then or having multiple gym or club memberships or spend a huge amount of money on high tech gadgets or spend on very expensive fashionable or stylish clothing or fitness gears, then please do not forget about your own body and it's well-being. Never hesitate to pay the genuinely required amount of fees to a genuine and worth guide or coach, who could be really helpful and necessary in your fitness journey. It is value for money.

- **Truth is Light and Light shows the way:** Be Genuine to your own self and to your coach always. Do not hide any information which your coach would require or might be important to help you in your fitness journey. Provide all necessary information and facts regarding your health, fitness and wellness condition very genuinely to your coach and make his/her work easy and this indirectly benefit you to achieve your target or desired results in less time.

Preparation to start your Fitness Routine

Starting a fitness routine can be a great step towards improving your physical health and overall well-being. Here are some steps that can help you prepare:

1. **Consult a healthcare professional:** If you have any pre-existing medical conditions or have not been active for a while, it's important to speak with a healthcare professional or an experienced fitness expert to get a clearance before starting any exercise program.

2. **Set realistic goals:** Decide what you want to achieve through your fitness routine, such as losing weight, building muscle, improving flexibility, or simply becoming more active. Make sure your goals are specific, measurable, attainable, relevant, and time-bound (SMART).

3. **Create a plan:** Develop a plan for your fitness routine, including what type of exercise you'll do, how often, and for how long. Make sure your plan fits into your schedule and is realistic for you to stick to.

4. **Get the right gear:** Proper clothing and footwear is important. Wearing comfortable and appropriate clothing and footwear can help you

perform better and stay injury-free. Choose clothing that is breathable and allows for a full range of motion.

a) **Shoes:** Make sure your shoes provide proper support and stability, for that purpose you should get, specifically the 'Wide Toe Box Shoes', because it helps to spread the toes wider and get a proper grip on the ground which leads to great stability and balance by staying in the most natural position and it also keeps you away from the painful structural change condition called, 'Banian' causes because of narrow toe box shoes or regular footwears.

In the legs' workouts for the exercise like, 'Squats' doing it barefoot could possibly the ideal and effective way. But in a gym where there are other people, using weights around you, it is recommended to use shoes for the safety purpose and to avoid any kind of accidental injury.

b) **Supporters (For Men): 'Langot' is the traditional supporter used in India for men, and it is used for the same purpose and works similar to the fancy Supporters which are been used**

nowadays, these fancy supporters were invented and used in western countries. In India 'Langot' was widely used since ancient times and it is a must, in the practice of traditional way of exercises such as Surya namaskar, Malla Khamb, yoga etc. If you have to play any traditional sport especially 'Kushti'. You cannot start the practice and preparatory exercises required for 'Kushti', without wearing a 'Langot'. Langot or **Supporters**, also known as athletic supporters or jockstraps, are specialized undergarments designed to provide support and protection to the male genitalia during physical activity. They typically consist of an elastic waistband, a protective pouch for the penis and testicles, and two straps that go around the buttocks to hold the pouch in place.

The primary purpose of supporters is to prevent injury and discomfort during exercise or sports that involve running, jumping, or sudden changes in direction. The supportive pouch holds the genitals snugly in place, reducing the risk of twisting or impact-related injuries, and the straps provide extra stability and prevent the pouch from shifting or slipping.

Supporters are commonly worn during high-impact activities such as running, soccer, football, basketball, and martial arts. They are also recommended for weightlifting and other forms of strength training, as they can help improve form and stability during heavy lifts.

To their injury-prevention benefits, supporters can also provide a more comfortable and secure fit for athletes during exercise. By holding the genitals in place and reducing friction and chafing, supporters can help reduce discomfort and distractions, allowing athletes to focus more fully on their performance.

In terms of fitness gear, supporters are often considered a basic essential for male athletes and are commonly included in workout and sports apparel packages. They can be purchased in a variety of styles and materials, including cotton, nylon, and spandex, and may be combined with other supportive garments such as compression shorts or tights for added protection and comfort.

It's importance to prevent inguinal hernia in men: An inguinal hernia is a common condition that occurs when part of the intestine protrudes through a weak spot or tear in the abdominal wall, specifically in the groin area. While both men and women can develop inguinal hernias, they are much more common in men, with an estimated 25% of men developing one in their lifetime.

One of the most effective ways to prevent inguinal hernias in men is through the use of supporters or athletic cups during physical activity. This is because inguinal hernias often occur as a result of excessive pressure on the abdominal wall, which can happen during activities such as lifting heavy weights, playing sports, or doing strenuous exercises. When the pressure in the abdominal cavity becomes too great, it can cause the intestines to push through the weakened area and create a hernia.

Wearing a Langot or supporter or athletic cup can help alleviate some of this pressure by providing additional support to the abdominal wall and the surrounding muscles. This can help prevent development of hernia(s) and reduce the risk of injury during physical activity. Supporters can also help to improve posture and reduce strain on the lower back, which can further reduce the risk of hernias. **And this proves how wise ancient Indians were, about their lifestyle and health, so that they added and maintained the necessary things by default to its culture and as an essential part of their lifestyle. That's why 'Langot' is still seem to be as an important aspect to be considered for playing this ancient sport, 'Kushti'. Ancient Indians, have created and designed their culture very strategically, systematically and scientifically with lots of sense, philosophy and wisdom. This proves, how Indians always have been living and leading the world with example.**

Other lifestyle factors can also help to prevent inguinal hernia(s) in men. Maintaining a healthy weight, practicing good lifting techniques, and avoiding activities that require repetitive and extreme straining, can help to reduce the risk of hernia(s).

And most importantly in the initial phase of the workouts as a beginner we should always focus on Strengthening and conditioning of core area which includes, Abdominal muscles, lower back muscles, side obliques, transverse abdominal sheet, and some part of hip muscles attached to pelvic joint internally. And also, **should avoid some intense stretches and advance poses or Asanas in Yoga, Power Yoga and Surya namaskar which could be risky at times considering few aspects.** Men who have a family history of hernia or who have already experienced a hernia (beginning phase) in the past, may also be advised to take additional precautions, such as avoiding heavy lifting or strenuous exercise and **focus more on core conditioning and strengthening exercises on regular basis, especially if they are starting their fitness routine after a long gap.**

Overall, the importance of preventing inguinal hernia(s) in men cannot be overstated. While hernias can often be repaired through surgery, they can be painful, uncomfortable, and can cause complications if left untreated. By taking simple steps such as Working on the core group muscles and strengthen them on a regular basis, but starting with simple and basic exercises and the with consistency progress gradually, wearing supporters and practicing good lifting techniques, men can greatly reduce their risk of developing inguinal (Specifically) hernia(s) and enjoy an active and healthier lifestyle.

c) **Sports Bra (For Women):** Sports bras are essential for women who engage in physical activities such as working out, running, or practicing sports. The following are some reasons why sports bras are important:

1. **Support:** During physical activities, breasts can bounce and move around, causing discomfort and pain. Sports bras are designed to provide support and prevent breast movement, reducing discomfort and preventing injuries.

2. **Comfort:** Sports bras are made from breathable materials that wick away moisture, keeping you comfortable and dry during physical activities. They are also designed to fit snugly, reducing chafing and irritation.
3. **Prevents Sagging:** Excessive bouncing and movement of the breasts can cause damage to the breast tissue, leading to sagging. Sports bras can help prevent this by minimizing breast movement during physical activities.
4. **Prevents Health Issues:** The lack of proper support during physical activities can lead to several health issues such as shoulder, back, and neck pain. Sports bras help to prevent these problems by providing proper support.
5. **Improves Performance:** Wearing a sports bra can improve performance by providing support and comfort, allowing you to focus on the activity at hand.

Overall, sports bras are essential for women who engage in physical activities. They provide support, prevent discomfort, reduce the risk of injuries, and improve performance. It is important to choose a sports bra that fits well and provides the right level of support for your body type and activity level.

But on the other hand, make sure that the sports bra or even the 'regular bra' in that matter, should never be too tight, because it may affect the efficiency and the overall work of lymph system in that particular area around breasts and cause damage to that particular area. If the bra is very tight then it restricts the lymphatic system, which can be called the drainage system of the body and is responsible for draining out the toxins from the muscles.

The lymphatic system is an important part of the human body's immune system. It is a network of vessels and organs that help remove waste, toxins, and other harmful substances from the body and fight off infections. The lymphatic system is located throughout the body, but its primary function in the chest area is to:

1. **Drain excess fluid:** The lymphatic vessels in the chest area collect excess fluid and waste products from the tissues and return them to the bloodstream. This helps to prevent swelling and edema (also known as swelling, is a medical condition in which an excess of fluid accumulates in the body's tissues, leading to the visible swelling of affected areas. This condition can occur in any part of the body, including the legs, ankles, feet, hands, and face, and is often

caused by an underlying health condition such as heart or kidney disease, circulatory disorders, liver disease, or certain medications. Edema can cause discomfort, pain, and limited mobility in the affected areas, and in severe cases, it can lead to skin ulcers or infections. Treatment of edema usually involves identifying and addressing the underlying cause of the condition, as well as lifestyle changes such as reducing salt intake, exercising regularly, and wearing compression garments. In some cases, medications may also be prescribed to help reduce swelling and manage the underlying condition.) in the chest and trunk area. From another point of view, swelling occurred due to different radiations around us, like Wi-Fi, mobile network, microwave etc. Also, everything around us carries certain amount and level of frequencies. 'Fabric', is one of the common and most important things in our daily usage, so its very important to use clothes made out of such fabric which carries a certain level of frequencies (Higher than the human body's frequencies) if in case the frequencies don't match (less than the human body's frequency) can lead to swelling/

inflammation or other complications. So, make sure that you choose the right size, so that it won't affect the work of lymphic system and if the Lymphic System works at its best then the swelling causing excessive fluid present in affected area or muscles will easily be carried out through this drainage system of the body.

2. **Absorb fats:** The lymphatic system in the chest area also absorbs fats and fat-soluble vitamins from the digestive system and transports them to the bloodstream.

3. **Fight infections:** The lymphatic system contains lymphocytes and other immune cells that help to identify and destroy foreign substances such as viruses and bacteria that enter the body.

4. **Transport immune cells:** The lymphatic vessels in the chest area also transport immune cells and antibodies throughout the body to fight infections and disease.

The lymphatic system plays a vital role in maintaining the health and wellbeing of the body, particularly in the chest and trunk area.

And if the lymphatic system gets affected then the toxins and dead cells and other debris gets accumulated in this area around the chest and this accumulation leads to swelling and pain. And if not worked on it in time may lead to formation of cancerous (carcinogenic) cells and if still ignored it may further turn out into **'Breast Cancer'**.

So, it's a humble request to all the ladies out there, please make sure that the selection of a bra shouldn't be done just to enhance your superficial looks on temporary basis, but also make sure that your comfort, internal health and well-being should be maintained and enhanced in long run and it should be taken in consideration on priority basis, always.

d) A pair of fresh socks: Always carry and wear an odourless, Fresh and clean pair of socks while going for your workouts.

e) Deodorant or Perfume: If it is known to you or anyone bring it to your notice about your body odour, then never ever forget to wear a deodorant of body spray or perfume with a decent and moderate fragrance to make yourself more presentable and hygienic.

f) Hand Towel/ Napkin: Always carry two Napkins or hand towels, one for wiping your own body and face. Other one to place on bench or mat which you will be using for any particular set of exercise or workout, also wipe the bench or mat once you are done with that particular set of exercise, using the same Napkin or Hand towel. This is very important in regards with the hygiene, discipline and gym etiquettes.

g) Water Bottle: While going to gym, always carry a clean water bottle filled with clean potable water, preferably metal (Copper), rather than a glass or plastic one.

h) Bath Towel, Body Soap or Shampoo: In case if you are going to take shower and if the shower and steam facility is available at your gym.

i) Comfortable Gym Bag: Make sure that your gym bag is comfortable to carry and it should be of a good size so that the above-mentioned things plus extra pair of clothing should get accommodate easily and it should not be much trouble for you to carry.

Invest in appropriate workout clothing and footwear that's comfortable and allows for full range of motion. Consider purchasing any necessary equipment such as dumbbells (in case of home-based workouts), resistance bands (Home based workouts and in case of rehab, strengthening, conditioning exercises), or a yoga mat (if required).

5. **Warm up and cool down:** Make sure to start each workout with a 5–10-minute warm-up to gradually increase your heart rate and prepare your muscles for exercise. After your workout, cool down with a light stretch or walk. Your foundation is the beginning of exercise journey and it is very important phase. So, don't underestimate the warm up and cool down part. Get habitual to it and most importantly learn the correct way and the right techniques with great details and follow, use it wisely always. Don't be lazy or don't feel shy to do the simplest forms of micro movements, know that they are an important part of your fitness plan/ program.

6. **Stay hydrated:** Drink plenty of water before, during, and after your workout to stay hydrated. Staying hydrated is crucial for performance and to prevent dehydration. You should drink sufficient and required quantity of water before, during, and after exercise to replace the fluids lost through sweating.

7. **Track your progress:** Keeping a record of your workouts and progress can help keep you motivated and on track. You can use a journal, app, or spreadsheet to log your workouts, weight, and other measurements.

Remember, it's important to listen to your body and progress at your own pace, without comparing or competing with anyone else. If you experience any pain or discomfort, stop and seek an expert's advice.

8. **Mix it up:** Doing a variety of exercises can help you prevent boredom and target different muscle groups. Consider incorporating strength training, cardio, stretching, and core exercises into your routine, but make sure that the choice of the exercises should always be done on the basis of my, **'4S' formula**. (**'4S' formula** stands for – **Safe, Simple, Suitable and Sustainable**).

9. **Find a workout buddy:** Having a workout partner can help keep you accountable and motivated. You can also motivate, support and help each other reach your fitness goals.

10. **Get sufficient sleep:** Sleep is important for physical recovery and overall health. Aim for 6-9 hours of sleep (might be different for different people) per night to ensure your body has sufficient time duration to recover after a workout.

11. **Fuel your body:** Eating a healthy, balanced diet is crucial for fuelling your workouts and supporting recovery. Make sure to eat required quantity of protein to support muscle growth

and repair. And plenty of fruits, vegetables, and whole grains for energy and nutrients.

12. **Stay positive:** Starting a fitness routine can be challenging, but it's important to stay positive and focus on the benefits. Celebrate your successes, no matter how small it is, and keep a growth mindset all the time.

By following these tips and being consistent with your fitness routine, you'll be well on your way to reaching your goals and improving your health and well-being.

Pre-requisites of Workout

There are a few things that are generally considered to be the prerequisites for a safe and effective workout:

1. **A clear mind:** Exercising with a clear mind and positive attitude can help you get the most out of your workout and can also help to reduce stress and anxiety.

2. **Safety considerations:** If you have any pre-existing medical conditions, it's important to talk to your doctor before starting a new exercise routine. If you're new to exercise, it's also important to start slow and progress gradually to reduce the risk of injury.

    A proper warm-up, hydration, appropriate clothing and footwear, a clear mind, and consideration of any safety concerns are important prerequisites for a workout.

3. **Goal setting:** Having specific, achievable goals can help you stay motivated and focused during your workout. Whether you want to improve your fitness level, lose weight, or build muscle, having clear goals can help you make the most of your time and effort.

4. **Good nutrition:** Eating a balanced diet that provides your body with the nutrients it needs

can help you perform better and recover faster from exercise. It's also important to eat enough to support your fitness goals and to fuel your workouts.

5. **Rest and recovery:** Allowing your body time to rest and recover is just as important as the workout itself. Over-training can lead to injury and burnout, so it's important to listen to your body and take rest days as needed.

6. **A suitable environment:** Creating a safe and suitable environment for your workout can help you focus and perform at your best. This may include access to a gym, suitable equipment, and a supportive workout partner or group.

7. **Professional guidance:** Seeking professional guidance from a certified personal trainer, physiotherapist, or other qualified fitness professional can help you achieve your goals faster and more safely. This can include help with developing an exercise plan, proper form and technique, and injury prevention.

Goal setting, good nutrition, rest and recovery, a suitable environment, and professional guidance are additional prerequisites that can help you get the most out of your workout.

Body Exercise Mechanism

Biological or Physical Exercise:

Physical exercise is **any bodily activity that enhances or maintains physical fitness and overall health and wellness**. But these needs to be done on regular basis and one can achieve higher level of fitness by constant efforts and progression in right direction, means by doing right and suitable exercises. Physical exercises can be different for different people depending up on certain factors. We generally think of physical exercise as activities that are undertaken for the main purpose of improving physical fitness which leads to overall health and wellness.

Mechanism of Exercise:

During physical exercise, requirements for oxygen and substrate in skeletal muscle are increased, as are the removal of metabolites and carbon dioxide. Chemical, mechanical and thermal stimuli affect alterations in metabolic, cardiovascular and ventilatory function in order to meet these increased demands. And with practice these consistently there is always a scope for improved ability and improved tolerance over the period of time.

Regular physical activity can improve your muscle strength and boost your endurance. Exercise delivers oxygen and nutrients to your tissues and helps your cardiovascular system work more efficiently. And when your heart and lung health improve, you have more energy to tackle daily chores.

When you do a moderate level exercise your body releases a Hormone called Endorphin, which gives a feeling of Happiness. It makes you feel good, but if you overdo any type of exercises for longer duration or do at a very high intensity and for longer time duration, then the body releases Stress hormone called 'Cortisol' (It is a hormone produced by the adrenal glands in response to stress, and it plays a key role in the body's stress response. During periods of physical stress, cortisol levels can rise in order to mobilize energy stores and help the body cope with the demands being placed on it. However, chronically elevated cortisol levels due to overtraining or excessive exercise can have negative effects on the body, including increased inflammation, decreased immune function, and impaired recovery.), that's why the exercises have to be at moderate levels of intensity and moderate time duration only. There is a saying 'Anything in excess can be poisonous.' So, one should always remember this and set the right and suitable limitations as per own body's understanding of abilities. This is how the body works, while it's in action to perform any physical exercise. We may count moderate to intense level physical works like Gardening, dish washing, sweeping, mopping, cooking, driving and so on, as physical exercise or biological exercise.

Precautions of Restarting after a long gap

Restarting a fitness routine after a long gap can be exciting, but it is important to take certain precautions to avoid injury and ensure that you are able to gradually build up your fitness level. Here are some precautions to keep in mind:

1. **Consult with an Experienced Fitness Expert/ Coach:** If you have any health conditions or concerns, it is important to consult with an Experienced Fitness Expert/ Coach before starting a new fitness routine. They can advise you on the best way to proceed, including any specific precautions or limitations you should be aware of.

2. **Understand and Analyse:** After a long break to your workouts, there are lots of unavoidable changes that may occur into your body internally or externally. Analyse and understand those changes and act accordingly. Make wise choices in selection of the exercises as per the current body conditioning. If you were a good athlete in past and stopped your exercise routine suddenly, then there are possibilities of the body to go into deconditioning phase. Even if you did

a good workout in past and stopped it suddenly and are currently into a sedentary lifestyle then also, we see a lot of changes in the body, like muscle loss, weakening of muscles, extra fat deposition, especially in the lower part of abdomen, waist area and hips area, also stiffness of muscles and joints, pain at times.

3. **Start slowly:** After a long gap, it can be tempting to dive right back into a challenging fitness routine. However, this can increase the risk of injury. Instead, start with low-impact activities and gradually increase the intensity and duration of your workouts over time.

4. **Warm up and cool down properly:** Warming up and cooling down are important for preventing injury and helping your body adjust to the physical demands of exercise. Start each workout with a 5–10-minute warm-up, such as light cardio or dynamic stretching, and end with a cool-down that includes stretching.

5. **Focus on form:** good form is essential for avoiding injury and getting the most out of your workouts. Pay attention to your posture and technique, and if you're unsure, consider working with a personal trainer or taking a class to learn proper form.

6. **Listen to your body:** If you feel pain or discomfort during a workout, stop and rest.

Don't push yourself too hard, especially if you are just starting out. It's better to take it slow and make progress gradually than to risk injury.

7. **Stay hydrated:** Staying hydrated is important for overall health, and it is especially important during physical activity. Drink water before, during, and after your workouts to help your body perform at its best.

8. **Variety:** Doing the same workout over and over again can lead to boredom and increase the risk of injury. Mix up your routine by incorporating different types of exercise, such as strength training, cardio, and stretching, to challenge your body in different ways and prevent boredom.

9. **Gradually increase intensity:** Gradually increasing the intensity of your workouts is key to avoiding injury and improving your fitness level. This can mean increasing the weight you're lifting, increasing the duration or intensity levels of your cardio workouts, or incorporating more challenging exercises.

10. **Recovery:** Rest and recovery are just as important as exercise. Give your body time to recover by taking at least one day off each week, and if you're feeling especially sore or tired, take an extra day or two off to allow your body to recover.

11. **Set realistic goals:** Setting realistic goals can help you stay motivated and on track. Rather than aiming to be in the best shape of your life in just a few weeks, set small, achievable goals that you can work towards over time.
12. **Consider working with a trainer:** If you're unsure about the best way to proceed with your fitness routine, consider working with a personal trainer. They can help you develop a safe and effective workout plan, and provide guidance and support as you work towards your goals.

By taking these precautions, you can restart your fitness routine in a safe and effective way, and avoid injury while building up your fitness level over time. And you can restart your fitness routine in a safe and effective way, and work towards a healthy, active lifestyle. Remember to be patient and consistent, and focus on making progress gradually over time.

Understanding Human Body in terms of Waves, Vibrations and Frequencies

The human body can be understood in terms of waves, vibrations, and frequencies in several ways.

One way to think about it is that the body is made up of atoms and molecules, which are constantly in motion and generate vibrations. These vibrations create patterns of energy that can be modelled as waves, and these waves have specific frequencies associated with them. The different frequencies of these waves are associated with different types of tissue and structures within the body, such as bones, muscles, and organs.

Another way to think about the body in terms of waves, vibrations, and frequencies is in terms of bioelectromagnetic fields. The human body generates electric and magnetic fields that are associated with its normal functions, such as nerve impulses and muscle contractions. These fields can be modelled as waves and have specific frequencies, which can provide information about the state of health of the body.

In the field of alternative medicine, there are theories that propose that certain frequencies and vibrations can be used to promote healing in the body. For example, in sound therapy, specific frequencies and vibrations of sound waves are used to balance and harmonize the body's energy. Similarly, in light therapy, specific frequencies and intensities of light are used to affect the body's energy and promote healing.

It is important to note that while the human body can be understood in terms of waves, vibrations, and frequencies, much of this understanding is still theoretical and not well supported by scientific evidence. Further research is needed to fully understand the relationship between the human body and these concepts.

The human body can also be understood in terms of waves, vibrations, and frequencies in terms of the way that it receives and processes information. For example, the body's sensory receptors, such as the eyes, ears, and skin, are designed to detect specific frequencies of light, sound, and pressure, which are then processed by the brain.

Similarly, the body's systems for communication and regulation, such as the nervous system and endocrine system, rely on waves and vibrations to carry signals and messages throughout the body. For example, nerve impulses are essentially electrical signals that propagate through the body as waves, and hormones are chemical signals that are produced and distributed by the endocrine glands.

In the field of medicine, various diagnostic techniques make use of waves, vibrations, and frequencies to obtain information about the body's functions. For example, ultrasound is a medical imaging technique that uses high-frequency sound waves to produce images of the inside of the body. Similarly, electroencephalography (EEG) measures the electrical activity of the brain and is used to diagnose conditions such as epilepsy. It is worth mentioning that there is ongoing research into the potential therapeutic applications of waves, vibrations, and frequencies in medicine. For example, researchers are exploring the use of low-frequency electromagnetic fields to promote healing in tissues and to treat conditions such as osteoarthritis. Similarly, researchers are investigating the use of sound and vibration therapy to alleviate pain and improve physical function in conditions such as fibromyalgia.

The human body can be understood in terms of waves, vibrations, and frequencies at various levels, from the molecular and cellular level to the systems level, and these concepts have important implications for our understanding of health and disease.

Electromagnetic Field of Human Body and Mother Earth

The human body, as well as the Earth, generates a complex electromagnetic field (EMF) that affects our physical and biological systems. In this context, electromagnetic field refers to a physical field produced by electrically charged objects that exerts a force on other charged objects within its field of influence. It can generate a weak electromagnetic field, primarily due to the flow of ions (positively and negatively charged particles) within our cells due to surroundings or due to not having a proper connection of human body with the plate of mother earth. The human body requires negatively charged ions from the atmosphere as well as from the earth plate to remain in the healthiest condition. This field can be affected by various factors, including our physical state, the presence of electric devices, even the things we use or we are surrounded by, carries certain number of frequencies and these frequencies can affect our body's EMF and the Earth's magnetic field and so on.

The Earth also generates a complex electromagnetic field, which is known as the geomagnetic field. This field is generated by the Earth's core, which is composed of molten iron and nickel, and it acts as a protective shield that helps to protect us from the harmful effects of solar radiation and cosmic particles.

The geomagnetic field also affects various natural phenomena, such as the migration patterns of birds and the growth patterns of certain plants, and it can also have an impact on our health and well-being. For example, some studies have suggested that changes in the Earth's magnetic field may be associated with an increased risk of migraines, depression, and other health conditions. To the other hand some cosmic energies also help human body update itself at cell levels or at DNA levels, if we come into contact with such energy fields, we generally feel chills, shivering, we may get goosebumps, we may feel a heavy head and sometimes we feel and hear the ringing in ears or at any particular side, most probably in the right ear. If we experience such things, know that our naturally inbuilt biological software is getting updated.

The electromagnetic fields generated by the human body and the Earth are complex and interrelated, and they play a role in many different aspects of our physical and biological systems. Understanding the impact of these fields on our health and well-being, and finding ways to minimize any negative effects, is an important area of research.

The Earth's atmosphere also generates a variety of electromagnetic fields, including the Schumann

Resonance, which is a global electromagnetic resonant cavity that exists between the surface of the Earth and the ionosphere. This resonance is produced by the interaction of lightning with the Earth's magnetic field, and it has been found to play a role in regulating our circadian rhythms, mood, and overall well-being.

The human body's electromagnetic field can also interact with other electromagnetic fields in our environment, such as those produced by electrical devices and power lines. This interaction can result in exposure to electromagnetic radiation, which has been linked to a variety of health problems, including cancer, fertility problems, and cognitive impairment.

To minimize exposure to harmful electromagnetic radiation, it is recommended to take steps to reduce exposure to electromagnetic fields, such as avoiding prolonged use of electronic devices, sleeping away from electrical appliances, and using shielding materials. It is also important to be mindful of the potential impact of electromagnetic fields on our health and well-being, and to be proactive about minimizing exposure to these fields whenever possible.

It's also worth noting that some people believe in the concept of "electromagnetic hypersensitivity," which is the idea that some individuals are more sensitive to electromagnetic fields and may experience physical symptoms as a result of exposure. While there is limited scientific evidence to support this idea, some studies have suggested a link between exposure to electromagnetic fields and various health problems, including headaches, fatigue, and sleep disturbances.

On the other hand, there is also evidence to suggest that exposure to certain types of electromagnetic fields may have therapeutic benefits. For example, low-frequency electromagnetic fields have been used in the treatment of various medical conditions, including depression, osteoporosis, and wounds.

In addition, there is a growing body of research on the use of electromagnetic fields for the treatment of various neurological conditions, such as Alzheimer's disease, Parkinson's disease, and stroke. This research is still in its early stages, and more studies are needed to determine the effectiveness and safety of these treatments. In that matter 'Med-beds' could be the future technology of the treatments for all the diseases.

The relationship between electromagnetic fields and human health is complex and not fully understood. While some studies suggest that exposure to electromagnetic fields may have harmful effects, others suggest that exposure to certain types of electromagnetic fields may have therapeutic benefits. Further research is needed to fully understand the impact of electromagnetic fields on our health and well-being.

The International Commission on Non-Ionizing Radiation Protection (ICNIRP) has established guidelines for exposure to electromagnetic fields from various sources, including power lines, wireless devices, and medical equipment. These guidelines are based on extensive research and are designed to protect the public from the potential health risks associated with exposure to electromagnetic fields.

However, it's also important to consider the context in which exposure to electromagnetic fields occurs. For example, exposure to electromagnetic fields from a single source, such as a cell phone, is typically much lower than the exposure from other sources, such as power lines or electrical appliances. Additionally, the duration and frequency of exposure can also play a role in the potential health risks associated with electromagnetic fields.

In conclusion, while exposure to high levels of electromagnetic fields can be harmful to our health, the vast majority of exposure levels that people experience in their daily lives are well within safe limits established by international health organizations. Nevertheless, it is still important to be mindful of potential health risks associated with exposure to electromagnetic fields, and to take steps to minimize exposure whenever possible.

Golden Ratio and Human Body Design

The Golden Ratio, also known as the Divine Proportion, is a mathematical concept that refers to a special number that appears frequently in nature, art, and design. It is approximately equal to 1.6180339887 and can be represented by the Greek letter Phi (Φ).

In design, the Golden Ratio is often used to create aesthetically pleasing compositions by dividing a space or an object into two parts in such a way that the ratio of the smaller part to the larger part is the same as the ratio of the larger part to the whole. This creates a harmonious and balanced arrangement that is pleasing to the eye.

Human body symmetry is another concept that is related to the Golden Ratio. The human body is often considered to be aesthetically pleasing when its various parts are in proportion to each other, and the Golden Ratio is sometimes used as a guide to achieve this balance. For example, the distance between the shoulder and hip is often said to be in the Golden Ratio to the distance from the hip to the knee.

It's important to note that while the Golden Ratio and human body symmetry are often discussed together, there is no scientific evidence to suggest that the human body is specifically designed to conform to the Golden Ratio. Nevertheless, the use of the Golden Ratio in design and the observation of its prevalence in nature have made it a popular concept in the fields of mathematics, art, and design.

The use of the Golden Ratio in design can be seen in a wide range of fields, including architecture, graphic design, web design, photography, and fashion. In architecture, the Golden Ratio has been used to design buildings, such as the Parthenon in Greece and the Notre-Dame Cathedral in France, that are considered to be aesthetically pleasing. In graphic design, the Golden Ratio can be used to determine the placement of elements on a page, such as text and images, to create a harmonious layout.

In web design, the Golden Ratio can be used to determine the placement of elements on a website, such as the header, sidebar, and footer, to create a visually appealing layout. In photography, the Golden Ratio can be used to determine the placement of objects in a frame to create a balanced composition. In fashion, the Golden Ratio can be used to determine the proportions of clothing items, such as the length of a skirt or the width of a tie, to create an aesthetically pleasing look.

It is worth mentioning that while the Golden Ratio is a useful tool for designers and artists, it is just one of many tools that can be used to create aesthetically pleasing designs. Ultimately, the goal of design is to create something that is visually appealing and functional, and the use of the Golden Ratio is just one way to achieve this. Some designers and artists feel that the strict adherence to the Golden Ratio can lead to overly formulaic designs, while others believe that it should be used as just one of many tools in a designer's toolkit. The use of the Golden Ratio in design is not limited to the visual arts. It has also been used in other fields, such as music and literature, to create harmonious and balanced compositions. For example, in music, the Golden Ratio has been used to determine the proportions of different elements, such as the lengths of musical phrases and the placement of beats, to create a pleasing rhythm. In literature, the Golden Ratio has been used to determine the proportion of different elements, such as the length of chapters and the number of paragraphs, to create a balanced and harmonious structure.

It is also worth noting that the Golden Ratio is just one of many mathematical concepts that have been used in design. Other mathematical concepts, such as the Fibonacci sequence and the Fibonacci spiral, are also frequently used to create aesthetically pleasing designs.

In conclusion, while the Golden Ratio is a popular tool in design, its use is not without controversy. Some designers and artists believe that it is a useful tool for creating aesthetically pleasing designs, while others believe that its strict adherence can lead to overly formulaic designs. The Golden Ratio has also been used in other fields, such as music and literature, to create harmonious and balanced compositions.

Understand Functioning of Human Body

Let's understand the base of the human body, which is a very complex combination of:

Visible Body – It is a Gross Physical Body, a combination of Bones, Muscles, Skin, Hairs, Internal Organs and so on. In physical body, length or height of the person, Different parts of the face including eyes (including its' colour), nose, lips, ears, hairs and skin (including it's colour), body structure or body type or body frame, body shape and size, this is the first look or we may call it as the first impression of the Physical body.

Invisible Body - We may consider it as Vibrational Bodies or Holographic bodies, these are the layers of bioelectromagnetic fields which have a certain range and these 3 bodies are Emotional, Psychological and Spiritual Body.

There are Five sheaths, which are very smartly designed and complement one another and keep a person alive. And by balancing all of them can lead to the benefits of Health and wellness in the most divine order.

- **Physical body:** This is obvious and gross body, it is made up of the skin, muscles, organs, blood, bones and different types liquids and fluids and so on. The tiny cells are the base of all the things mentioned above.
- **Astral body:** Our astral bodies are our way of feeling pleasure or pain.
- **Causal body:** The casual body, aka the seed body, is our blueprint of the gross and subtle bodies.

And the Ayurvedic types (also called the 'Doshas') are Pitta, Vata, and Kapha.

Ayurveda describes 7 basic body-types:

- **Vata dominant.**
- **Pitta dominant.**
- **Kapha dominant.**
- **Vata/Pitta (pitta/vata) – bidoshic body-type.**
- **Pitta/Kapha (kapha/pitta) – bidoshic body type.**
- **Kapha/Vata (vata/kapha) – bidoshic body type.**
- **Vata/Pitta/Kapha – tridoshic body type which is rare.**

If we Consider Ayurveda then following are the types of physical bodies in general.

'Pitta' represents 'Mesomorph' – Medium/Average Body Structure/Frame.

'Vata' represents 'Ectomorph' – Thin/Lean Body Structure/Frame.

'Kapha' represents 'Endomorph' – Thick/Large Body Structure/Frame.

Apart from the physical and visible bodies including the bones, muscles, different organs, blood, veins, nerves ayurveda mentioned way more details about the different fluids, liquids (Chemicals and hormones) and Air/ Gases (Prana Vayu) of different densities actively working at different locations/ parts in the body and the density or the type of Gas (Vayu) defines it's functioning and location in the body. These gases are actually very important as, the air for a tyre or balloon. If the air comes out of the tyre or balloon then the tyre or the balloon is useless. It is the air which serves the actual purpose of the Tyre or Balloon to put the 'life' into it. Without this 'Prana' (air) it is lifeless.

In General, following are the actual body types categorized according to the physical structure:

Most people are unique combinations of the three body types: **ectomorph, mesomorph, and endomorph**. Ectomorphs are long and lean, with little body fat, and little muscle.

Understanding the different physiological body types can give your insight into how it works best. The hormonal body types are Adrenal, Thyroid, Liver and Ovary, the structural types are **Ectomorph, Endomorph and Mesomorph**.

And from the Fitness and Health Prospective, you don't have just a Physical body (Whenever there is something about Health and Fitness, people generally just think about Physical Body, especially when it's about 'Physical Fitness', which covers strength, stamina and flexibility etc.), but you also have Emotional Body, Psychological/ Mental Body, Spiritual Body and Etheric Body as well. Now let's explore what these bodies are all about? and How they all are important and inter linked with each other in regards to your health and fitness?

As we see different colours, we can hear different sounds around us. We can feel the touch, we can see, we can hear, we can smell and we can feel the taste and also able to differentiate in between them (taste, sound, colour etc). The Human physical body have senses and they are linked to certain frequencies and it has a limit, we could reach to very limited frequencies. Especially in the day light human eyes can see maximum number of colours. As we know there are different sound frequencies/waves, similarly there are different colours and every colour carries a frequency. And these frequencies are not just limited to sound and colour and other senses. But everything present in this universe carries a particular or multiple frequency. A dog can smell Hormones present inside human body; they say Dogs can smell your Fear. But humans can't, they don't have that ability or they are not able to resonate with that particular frequency of that particular sense. Bats can't see, but they can hear the sound frequencies which human can't. Similarly, an X-Ray machine can capture the image of human body showing internal organs, bones etc. which we cannot see with normal eyes. After pressing a button, we can see the bulb light on, spreading light in a dark room, but do we see the 'current' passing through the wire and reach to the bulb? NO, we can't see the current, but definitely feel it, many of us must have experienced this electric current or shock at some point in our lives. Same way we can feel the hot and cold water, but cannot see the changes happened in the water body at the molecular levels, we can surely tell Hot and cold temperatures surely exists. And these are many such examples around us which we experience in our day today life. Being a human, we carry a great potential and at the same time, we are fortunate enough to raise our consciousness and awareness levels, but unfortunately, we possibly could limit our own selves from exploring our own potential. God has given us that neutrality which I guess no other entities have. I guess 'Human Beings' must be the greatest experience done by God, and it is a perfect representation of 'Yin and Yang'. The universe has probably millions of different frequencies may be more and so as Dimensions too. And every frequency or a set of combined frequencies creates a dimension and this dimensional field's area depends on the frequency itself. And know that these all frequencies are connected, everything in the universe is interlinked and interconnected.

Every Human Body has its own electromagnetic field, similarly it creates wavelengths of different colour frequencies of light. But these can't be seen with eyes. And these lights are also called as aura. And the power of the Aura depends on the conscious levels or the higher frequencies the person resonates in. This higher state can be achieved by multiple things, but the most important part is food, rich in vital nutrients, especially minerals, plants create its own food by photosynthesis and live it's healthy life, they get their energy from the sunlight, emitted by the direct source of energy 'SUN'. In case of humans we are considering our body on quantum system level, and by not considering the physical body only, but other bodies as well, we can utilise the energy of the lights received from the Source 'SUN', directly (absorbed through skin) or indirectly (In the form of Food Consumed – Fruits and Vegetables, especially plant based – where the energy/light is stored in the form of vitamins and minerals, Dairy – especially by the consumption of Cow's Milk, Surya Ketu Naadi (Surya Ketu Nerve) Present in the Hump of the cow when it comes in direct contact with sunlight, it absorbs all the positive energies and radiations and nutrients from the sunlight and produces GOLD Salt in the blood. Most of these GOLD salts are present in the Milk and Urine of the cow. And these GOLD salts have great medicinal properties and can cure many diseases. 'Gir' Cow (Mostly Found in the region of Gujrat, India) and other local (desi) Cows (Original and Pure Breeds) of Indian origin are found with this unique property.

Connect and energize yourself to the nature through basic elements

Our body is made up of 5 elements and we need to be connected with these elements to keep ourselves energised and charged to achieve and maintain the greatest divine level of Fitness, Health and Wellness. We need to connect with these five elements through the nature:

Water:

Sun Charged Water.

Water is very important for all living organisms. As we have seen above how Sunlight plays an important role for animal like cow, Similarly Sunlight is our main source of energy. Sunlight is the main element from which all living beings get their energy in the form of different colours and frequencies. These frequencies help us purify and get charged and energized.

Water and sunlight could be a great potential combination for the biological function of living beings at cell levels and it's natural systems. We store water in plastic tanks, bottles nowadays. Mostly the pipes are rustic and dirty from inside which carries the water. As a result, water loses all its energy and life and turns out to be 'dead'. Water becomes dead as soon as it disconnects from nature. In addition to this, many of us store water in plastic bottles, in summers many people refrigerate the water bottles and so on. Sun is original source of energy and sunlight bring this life energy to earth. Sunlight is the most important factor for Human health.

When sunlight falls upon water, it changes its molecular structure to convert it from DEAD WATER to LIVING WATER. At the point when we expend this sun-charged water, a similar life power is moved into our body and is utilized to heal our tissues and cells. This is very important for the people who live in Metro cities and small cities where main source of water supply is the trap of pipe line and maximum number of people, by default store the water in the Plastic Tanks, because of the system.

When water absorbs the sunlight, it develops a charge from the sunlight. Sun-charging water brings life back to water after it loses its aliveness. The UV rays in the sunlight can tear apart the microbes to make water safe. Light and heat oxidizes the water and infuse the water with natural benefits from Sun and Earth.

SUN CHARGED WATER BENIFITS

Sun charged water is revitalising and gives energy. It's consumption with herbs or medicines, makes healing faster with least side effects.

Major benefits are as follows:

- Increased energy levels.
- Creates rejuvenated feelings and Sense of well-being.
- Heals damages happened at cellular level.
- Clears urine and makes inner body more alkaline.
- Helps to maintain a good health of skin, skin becomes clear and increases glow.
- Good for the eye health and sight.
- It is anti-viral, anti-fungal, and anti-bacterial.

PROCEDURE TO MAKE SUN CHARGED WATER:

- Take fresh potable water in a shallow earthen pot or a glass container with broad surface area (avoid plastic container).
- Place the pot outside (on bare earth or rock or on cement) in direct sunlight. Do not place it on grass or sand.
- Cover this pot with a thin muslin cloth to prevent dirt entering water. Tie the muslin cloth to the pot using a rope or string.

- Keep the container in direct sunlight for around 5-7 hours, preferably in the morning at around 7-8 AM.

- Collect this charged water in your water dispenser and drink within 24 hours.

- Do not refrigerate this, sun charged water.

Sun Gazing: Sungazing is an ancient technique used to achieve benefits of physical, mental and spiritual enhancement. But it is very important that the technique of Sun gazing should be done in an accurate way. It should be done only at the time of Sun rise and Sun set. The beneficial effects of sungazing after receiving the direct sun rays through eyes, enter in to 3rd eye or pineal gland and it gets decalcify. Humans are 'light beings' and the 'light codes' coming from the sunlight moves through our eyes and charge the hypothalamus track and stimulate the 'Pineal Gland'. These light codes, apart from charging our body, are also encoded with the information and keys to unlock the dormant DNA within our body vessel. Unlocking our DNA is the key to access to our 'Etheric Body' and get connected to the 'Ether' present in the atmosphere and in to the entire universe, in short getting connected to nature and the universe.

The sunrays enter through the cornea and stimulate the Pituitary Gland and Pineal Gland, which helps to decalcify the brain and at the same time having the similar positive effect which we get after doing Yoga and Meditation. And this knowledge is commonly known in all cultures. Our ancestors knew that gazing directly at the sun, during sunrise and sunset has incredible benefits and a great positive impact on one's health. Since there are zero Ultra Violate (UV) rays at these times. And gazing sun at sunrise or at sunset your eyesight is not only undamaged but known to be improved in a great extent.

The Pineal Gland is a Light receptor. The brain is able to know to heal the body, at any stage of illness (spontaneous remissions). Light has played a central role in the treatment of many conditions, e.g. mood disorders, insomnia, anxiety, depression, PTSD (Post-Traumatic Stress Disorder), tumours, compulsive and mental disorders, the range of application is unlimited. Sunlight and darkness trigger the release of hormones in your brain. Exposure to sunlight is thought to increase the brain's release of a hormone called serotonin.

Precautions:

- Practice this only in recommended safe hours or time zone i.e. Only at the time of Sunrise and Sunset.

- Remove all kinds of obstacles like sun glasses or specs or lenses between the sun and your eyes, to enhance the benefits by multiple times.

- Never look at the sun via a telescope, camera, binoculars or a glass etc.

- Initially start with small, means start with short duration of time to avoid damage to the retina of eyes, with consistency and regular practice you may increase the time duration.

- If it hurts your eyes or feel any kind of sensation or pain or itchy sensation, then stop immediately.

It is never been recommended to gaze at the sun apart from these two ideal times and without any precautions for the purpose of safety of your eyes.

Benefits of Sungazing: The Sun is the force of all life by following this method of staring at it infuses the body with large amount of energy.

- Improved eyesight.
- Enhanced Vitality.
- Increased Energy.
- Supplies vitamin D.
- Improves immune system.

- Reduces Stress.
- Supplies nutrients to the brain.
- Increases your inner strength.
- Encourages a positive mindset.
- Lessens unnecessary appetite, reduces hunger cravings.
- Increased self-confidence.
- Increases Health, Longevity and Spiritual wellbeing.
- Boosts production of melatonin and serotonin hormones.
- Stimulation of Pineal Gland.
- Increases the actual size of Pineal Gland.
- Reducing and releasing of mental and physical blockages.
- Stress relief.

These are the benefits of Sun gazing on regular basis.

Natural Sources of Water are filled with essential nutrients.

Natural sources of potable water refer to sources of water that can be safely consumed without any treatment or purification. Here are some examples of natural sources of potable water and their nutritional values and benefits:

1. **Springs:** Springs are natural sources of water that emerge from the ground. They are usually clean and clear, and the water is rich in minerals such as calcium, magnesium, and potassium. Drinking spring water can help improve bone health, regulate blood pressure, and prevent kidney stones. Spring water is typically rich in minerals such as calcium, magnesium, potassium, and sodium. These minerals are essential for maintaining healthy bones, regulating blood pressure, and supporting nerve and muscle function. Calcium and magnesium are particularly important for strong bones, while potassium and sodium help regulate fluid balance in the body.

2. **Wells:** Wells are another natural source of potable water. The water from wells is usually free from contaminants and is rich in minerals such as iron and calcium. Drinking well water can help improve digestion, prevent anaemia, and strengthen teeth and bones. Well water can contain a variety of minerals depending on the geological makeup of the area. Common minerals found in well water include calcium,

iron, magnesium, and manganese. These minerals are important for various functions in the body, such as supporting bone health, aiding in digestion, and improving immune function.

3. **Rivers:** Rivers are natural sources of water that flow through the landscape. The water from rivers is usually clear and clean, but it may contain some contaminants. However, if you drink water from a river that is in a pristine area, you can benefit from the natural minerals and nutrients present in the water. Rivers can contain a range of minerals, depending on the source of the water and the surrounding environment. Generally, river water contains minerals such as calcium, magnesium, and potassium, as well as trace minerals like copper, zinc, and selenium. These minerals are essential for maintaining good health and preventing nutrient deficiencies.

4. **Lakes:** Lakes are natural bodies of water that are fed by streams, rivers, and rainwater. The water from lakes is usually clean, but it may contain some pollutants. Drinking water from a lake that is not contaminated can provide essential minerals such as calcium, magnesium, and sodium. Like rivers, the mineral content of lake water can vary depending on the source of

the water and the surrounding environment. However, lake water is generally rich in minerals such as calcium, magnesium, sodium, and potassium, as well as trace minerals like zinc and selenium, similar to river waters.

5. **Rainwater:** Rainwater is another natural source of potable water. It is pure and free from contaminants. Drinking rainwater can help improve digestion, boost immunity, and promote healthy skin. Rainwater is naturally pure and free from contaminants. However, it typically contains very low levels of minerals and nutrients, as it does not come into contact with the earth's mineral deposits. Nevertheless, drinking rainwater can still provide some benefits, as it can help to flush toxins from the body and promote healthy digestion. (But nowadays there are risk factors involved and the rain waters could possibly, be contamination or added chemicals due to the technologies used for artificial rains in many locations around the world).

Natural sources of potable water provide essential minerals and nutrients that are beneficial for our overall health and well-being. However, it is important to note that natural sources of water may contain contaminants, so it is important to ensure that the water is safe for consumption before drinking it. These natural sources of potable water can be an excellent source of essential minerals and nutrients that are important for maintaining good health. However, the nutritional content of these waters can vary depending on the source and the surrounding environment. It is important to be aware of the specific mineral content of the water you are drinking, and to ensure that it is safe and with most effective and beneficial for consumption.

Earth:

Earthing/ Grounding: Walking barefoot on natural surfaces has several benefits for our feet, body, and mind. Here are some of the benefits in detail:

1. **Improved foot strength:** Walking barefoot allows the muscles, tendons, and ligaments in our feet to work harder, leading to stronger feet and ankles. This can help improve balance and stability, reduce the risk of injury, and make daily activities such as standing and walking more comfortable. It also helps in improved movements and micromovements of the muscles present at the bottom of our feet and which directly gets connected to the surface of the earth plate. Waking with shoes or foot wears on, can restrict these micromovements of the muscles present at the sole, and because of lack of movements on regular basis these muscles

can become inactive, eventually stiff and muscle loss also can happen in some cases and further leads to pain in overall sole, burning sensation or develop into heel pain.

2. **Better proprioception:** Proprioception is the ability to sense the position, movement, and force of our body parts. Walking barefoot on different natural surfaces provides a variety of sensory information to the feet, improving our proprioceptive abilities. This can help us become more aware of our body and movements, leading to better balance, coordination, and posture.

3. **Enhanced circulation:** Walking barefoot on natural surfaces stimulates the nerve endings in our feet, which can improve blood flow and circulation throughout the body. This can help reduce inflammation, boost immunity, and promote healing.

4. **Reduced stress:** Walking barefoot on natural surfaces can have a calming effect on the mind and body. This is partly due to the release of endorphins, which are natural painkillers and mood boosters. Additionally, being in nature and connecting with the earth can help reduce stress, anxiety, and depression.

5. **Improved alignment:** Walking barefoot on natural surfaces requires us to adjust our gait and posture to the uneven terrain, which can help improve our alignment and reduce the risk of joint pain or injury. This can also help strengthen the muscles in our legs, hips, and back, leading to better overall health and wellness.

There are different natural surfaces and they can provide unique benefits for our feet and body. Here are some examples:

1. **Sand:** Walking barefoot on sand requires the muscles in our feet and ankles to work harder to maintain balance and stability. The shifting surface also provides a massage-like effect, which can help improve circulation and reduce tension in the feet.

2. **Grass:** Walking barefoot on grass can provide a cushioned surface that is gentle on the feet and joints. It can also help improve balance and coordination, as the uneven terrain requires us to adjust our gait and posture.

3. **Dirt:** Walking barefoot on dirt can be grounding and help reduce stress and anxiety. It can also provide a natural exfoliation for the feet, helping

to remove dead skin cells and promote healthy skin.

4. **Rocks:** Walking barefoot on rocks can provide a reflexology-like experience, stimulating various pressure points in the feet and promoting overall health and wellness. It can also help improve balance and strengthen the muscles in the feet and ankles.

Walking barefoot on different natural surfaces can provide a range of benefits for our feet, body, and mind. It can improve foot strength, enhance proprioception, boost circulation, reduce stress, improve alignment, and more. By exploring different natural surfaces, we can discover new ways to connect with the earth and promote our overall health and well-being.

Grounding may have a number of other potential health benefits, like:

1. **Reducing inflammation:** Grounding has been found to reduce inflammation in the body, which is a contributing factor to many chronic health conditions, including arthritis, heart disease, and cancer.

2. **Improving sleep:** Grounding has been shown to improve the quality of sleep by promoting relaxation and reducing stress.

3. **Reducing stress and anxiety:** Grounding has been found to reduce levels of the stress hormone cortisol and increase feelings of calmness and well-being.

4. **Boosting immune function:** Some studies suggest that grounding may help to boost immune function by reducing inflammation and oxidative stress in the body.

5. **Improving cardiovascular health:** Grounding has been shown to improve blood flow, lower blood pressure, and reduce the risk of heart disease.

6. **Reducing pain:** Grounding has been found to reduce pain in individuals with chronic pain conditions, such as fibromyalgia and osteoarthritis.

7. **Improving mood:** Grounding has been shown to improve mood and reduce symptoms of depression.

8. **Improving energy levels:** Grounding has been found to improve energy levels and reduce fatigue.

9. **Enhancing athletic performance:** Some athletes use grounding as part of their training

regimen, as it has been shown to improve athletic performance and reduce recovery time.

10. **Supporting healthy aging:** Grounding may help to slow down the aging process by reducing inflammation and oxidative stress in the body.

This is how we get connected with earth plate and get energized. Earth plate is our body's charger, so we need to get connected with it barefoot very often to keep our body battery fully charged and to function at optimum levels in day today life.

Air:

Fresh and Pure Air:

The element of air is an essential component of the human body. It plays a vital role in maintaining life and health. Here are some reasons why air is crucial for the human body:

1. **Breathing:** The most obvious importance of air is that it is the primary component of the air we breathe. Oxygen is necessary for cellular respiration, which is the process by which our bodies convert food into energy. Without oxygen, our cells would not be able to function, and we would die.

2. **Circulation:** The air we breathe also helps to circulate blood throughout our bodies. The

oxygen we inhale is transported to our tissues and organs by our blood, while carbon dioxide, a waste product of cellular respiration, is carried away from our tissues and expelled through our lungs.

3. **Cooling:** Air helps to regulate body temperature. When we breathe, we exhale warm air, which helps to cool our bodies. This is why we often breathe heavily when we are hot or exercising.

4. **Immune function:** Air plays a role in our immune function. The cells of our immune system rely on oxygen to function properly. When we inhale, we take in oxygen, which our immune cells use to destroy harmful bacteria and viruses.

5. **Mental health:** Air is also important for our mental health. Breathing deeply and slowly can help to calm our minds and reduce stress and anxiety.

The element of air is critical to the human body for a range of reasons, from providing the oxygen needed for cellular respiration to supporting immune function and mental health.

Oxygen and Pranayam:

Oxygen is essential for our survival, and pranayama is an ancient yogic practice that involves controlling the breath to improve overall health and well-being. Here are some of the ways oxygen and pranayama are important for our health:

1. **Oxygen is necessary for cellular respiration:** Our cells need oxygen to produce energy through cellular respiration. Without oxygen, our cells cannot function properly, and our organs and tissues can suffer damage.

2. **Pranayama can improve lung function:** Pranayama practices, such as deep breathing exercises, can help improve lung function by increasing the amount of oxygen we inhale and improving the efficiency of our respiratory system.

3. **Improved circulation:** By breathing deeply and consciously, pranayama can help to improve circulation throughout the body, including the delivery of oxygen to our cells and tissues.

4. **Stress reduction:** Pranayama can help to reduce stress and anxiety by activating the parasympathetic nervous system, which induces relaxation and reduces stress hormones.

5. **Improved immune function:** Oxygen is essential for the functioning of the immune system, and pranayama has been shown to enhance immune function by increasing oxygen levels in the body.

6. **Improved mental clarity and focus:** Pranayama practices can help to calm the mind and improve mental clarity and focus.

Oxygen is essential for our survival, and pranayama is an effective way to improve lung function, reduce stress, enhance immune function, and improve mental clarity and focus. Incorporating regular pranayama practices into our daily routines can have numerous benefits for our overall health and well-being.

Ether:

'Ether' is present in the atmosphere and in to the entire universe. Simple explanation about 'Ether' is that it connects everything with everything. It holds everything in the universe and keeps it in its original place. If it is been removed, everything in the entire universe will collapse. It is also called as the 'God Particle'. 'Ether' is also known as a divine form of 'Water', which is present everywhere and commonly known as 'Aakash' or 'Space'. We generally think 'space' is empty, but it is filled with 'Ether'.

In the universe, the concept of ether has been largely replaced by the understanding of the fabric of space-time in the framework of general relativity. According to this theory, space-time is a dynamic structure that can be warped by the presence of matter and energy. This has been supported by numerous observations and experiments, including the bending of starlight by the gravitational field of the Sun during a solar eclipse.

In the human body, the concept of "ether" is not recognized by modern scientific understanding of physiology. The term "ether" has been used historically to refer to a hypothetical substance that was believed to fill the universe and provide a medium for the transmission of light and other forms of electromagnetic radiation. However, this concept has been abandoned in modern physics, and the properties of light and electromagnetic radiation are now understood in terms of the behaviour of particles and fields. In some spiritual and holistic healing traditions, the term "ether" may be used to refer to an energy or life force that is believed to flow through the body and influence health and wellbeing. However, these concepts are not recognized by mainstream scientific understanding of the human body and its functions.

Even though we are trapped in the physical body, our soul remains the same for eternity, just changing the bodies like clothes and as per our karmic actions and reactions. Our soul carries the same energy which it has received from our creator, god or nature or universe whatever we may believe in. The core energy remains the same in every form of physical body we wear and that core is the God particle or we may call it Ether. It connects everything with everything. It could be present anywhere and everywhere. And our soul energy is a signature form of this universal energy.

As our soul energy remains the same, it carries the same frequencies of energy without our consciousness. Similarly, most of us might be knowing that, every word carries certain frequencies and energies. And that's the reason why too emotional people (rooted to their soul through their heart chakra) have certain level of consciousness. Such kind of people can't take it, if someone try to bully them or use bad words against them, they get emotional, they might even cry or become too angry at times. The reason behind it could possibly be that somewhere deep down into their heart and soul, they must be carrying the frequencies in the form of knowledge or memories or the effect of the frequencies and energies created by using such words. And this is the reason why we should never ever bully or curse or use bad or negative words towards anyone ever in our life. It will definitely put you into a karmic reaction cycle unknowingly.

Words are really powerful and carry tremendous number of energies either positive or negative. And the choice of selection of the words depends completely upon us. That's why our choice of words should always be wise and then only the energies carried by these words would be supporting and helpful not only to others but also for the person using them. This is the reason why Prayers, Blessings, Gratitude and Affirmations play an important role in Human life, in the nature and in the entire universe. All of the above mentioned are the powerful tools or energies packed in the form of vibrational frequencies or the words. And it completely depends up on us how we use it, whether to break the world or to make the world. In Indian ancient texts, the unimaginable importance of the 'Mantras' is explained in many situations and it is nothing else but the real power of words. The words we use can be used as a weapon to harm someone or as a miraculous medicine to heal someone. Take my words, that words can change our lives as they carry the power and the 'Universal energy' which means 'Etheric energy'.

'Ether' plays an important role in the history of science and philosophy; it is not recognized as a fundamental component of the human body or the universe by modern scientific understanding.

Beyond Imagination

Metaphysical, Holographic Bodies, Electromagnetic Energy Field bodies and much more, beyond our imagination is our 'Quantum Reality'.

The theory of the Human Body with visible body and invisible bodies. The gross physical body structures and the holographic or metaphysically present energy fields of our own reality, but everyone is not aware of it. So, we have our multiple realities present at the same time and it can be related to Quantum Mechanics or Quantum Physics.

As we consider the aspects of Fitness which we can actually feel. If we feel the awareness about our fitness and health, our consciousness about our wellbeing levels up and we become awakened about the process of achieving the Health, Fitness and wellness in the great divine order.

Scientists nowadays are very proud of their **Artificial Intelligence** (A.I.) technologies but, Human Beings can achieve the Greatest **Awakened Intelligence** (A.I.), This is God's gift given to human beings in a secretive way, we need to find out and explore it using the immense powers of our sub conscious mind. This A.I. can create miracles, solve mysteries of universe. Human Body is a Genius Design, combination of all forms of sciences i.e., Physics, Quantum Physics, Engineering, Mechanical Engineering, Chemistry, Biology, Microbiology, Physiology, Kinesiology, Psychology and there are possibilities that there must be many more technologies used and we are not aware of their existence, in fact our brain might not have the capacity to understand such kind of technologies.

Physical Body: This is the gross, physical structure with certain symmetry. This decides shape, size and overall physical look of a person and this is the first impression of the personality of any person.

Mental/Psychological Body: This all about the thoughts, intelligence, understanding and to act or express one self, based on the thoughts depending upon the situation. This is an important and complex body which plays an important role in one's character or personality and the very basic function of decision making.

Emotional Body: This is about Emotions and Expression without the interference of Mental Body. This is also situation based. Your emotions are expressed differently at different situations. Emotions could be also different towards different personalities or people around us. Strongest emotions could make you strongest or weakest at times or as per the situations. So, you need to have a great balance or control over your emotions in that case you need to allow your Mental/

Psychological Body to interfere and make decisions. These emotions are responsible for the secretion or releasing some type of hormones in different locations of the body and this pays very important role in the functionality of the physical body.

Spiritual Body: The Spiritual body is related to one's faith or belief. Being Spiritual or Faithful or Believer makes you more positive. So, in short being more spiritual means having a great balance and coordination in between your Mental and Emotional Bodies. Which helps you to have good control over these two bodies individually as well as in common. And this makes you wise, helps you to gain more wisdom. And helps you not just in making good decisions, but wise decisions in all situations and at all levels.

Spiritual View:

From the perspective of Spiritual View and Yogic Practices, 7 Chakras (6 Chakras - Wheels, it has a certain electromagnetic field around them and resonating at a particular Frequency on an individual basis) Present Inside the Body, aligned at a specific location in our Spine and 1 Chakra is Present just above the head similar to a crown, but it is like floating, not attached with the body).

Root/ Muladhara Chakra: The Base Chakra is called Root Chakra. It's colour is Red. The frequency of this

Chakra can be blocked by the emotional frequency of fear. This chakra deals with survival and Grounding. This chakra is located at the base of the spine, at tail bone.

Sacral/ Swadhishthana Chakra: The Sacral chakra is located above the Root Chakra, at the Naval Region. It's colour is Orange. The frequency of this chakra could be blocked by the emotional frequency of Guilt. This chakra deals with Sexuality and Passion.

Solar Plexus/ Manipura Chakra: The Solar Plexus Chakra is located above the Sacral Chakra, at the centre of the abdominal region. It's colour is Yellow. The frequency of this chakra could be blocked by the emotional frequency of Shame. This chakra deals with Confidence and Intuitions.

Heart/ Anahata Chakra: The Heart Chakra is located above Solar Plexus Chakra, at Chest Region. It's Colour is Green. The frequency of this chakra could be blocked by the emotional frequency of Grief. This Chakra deals with Love and Compassion.

Throat/ Vishuddha Chakra: The Throat Chakra is located above Heart Chakra, at Throat Region. It's colour is Blue. The frequency of this chakra could be blocked by the mental frequency of Lies. This chakra deals with Expression and Creativity.

Third Eye/ Ajna Chakra: The Third Eye Chakra is located above the Throat Chakra, in the Brain exactly in between the eyebrows at the forehead region. It's Colour is Indigo. The frequency of this chakra could be blocked by the psychological frequency of Illusion. This chakra deals with Psychic Ability and Insight.

Crown/ Sahasrar Chakra: The Crown Chakra is located above the Third Eye Chakra, above the Head. It is not attached with the body or head and it is like in a floating state above head. It's colour is Violet. The frequency of this chakra can be blocked by the emotional and psychological frequencies of attachment and ego. This chakra deals with Cosmic Energy and Connection with Universe and the Creator itself.

As I mentioned earlier, everything is interlinked and interconnected. Every aspect or part of the body or bodies can affect each other. Or they can react to each other's action, also depends up on each other. As long as we have a great inner-standing about the balance and rise to the higher frequencies we could possibly explore different realms and dimensions for the betterment of own self, as well as nature, our surroundings, other human beings or other beings who are part of the universe and the entire universe which leads us all towards the greater connection with the creator itself.

And these things, including the types of bodies and their aspects on an individual level which already exist parallelly, could possibly be known to different people with different names and different understanding depending upon multiple factors like their location, language, belief system, culture, tradition, teachings and so on.

Base /5 Elements' Body: Aetheric body is the combination of the 5 elements present in the nature/universe. These 5 elements are also present inside our body. And this is the bridge to connect us with the nature/universe. Air, Fire, Water, Earth and Space/ Ether. These are all present in different forms and at different locations inside the body.

Different types of Air and Gases are responsible for different functions inside the body at different internal organs and different location.

Similarly, the element of Fire is also present in a different format or in the form of energy in the intestine and helps in the function of digestion.

Water is an essential part as well, it is present in almost every liquid, fluid and hormones/ chemicals in the body at different locations and at different organ functions and responsible for different functions or carry out different activities inside the body.

Earth is also one of the important elements and is present in the body in a particular format and carry out different functions at different locations inside the body.

And Space which is present everywhere, it connects everything though it is full of emptiness. This is also an important element present inside and outside of the body and it is the connector for everything. This means there is everything but nothing. And when we see through the quantum aspect at quantum level, it proves the theory of quantum physics. Everything exists parallelly.

Apart from this Oxygen, Hydrogen, Carbon, Nitrogen, Calcium, Phosphorous, Sodium, Potassium, Magnesium, Sulphur, Chlorine is also present in the human body as different elements and metals.

As I mentioned, different people know these things with different name or with a different aspect or approach, here is a good example. In Chinese ancient medicinal science, they count Fire, Water, Earth, Wood and Metal as the 5 elements.

There are different proportions of 5 elements inside the Human body.

3-5% Fire, 5-8% Air, 10-15% Earth, 70-75% Water approximately, And the Ether is the remaining part but it's proportion may fluctuate or change depending up on the situation or depending up on the individual body and different health condition. Each element is responsible for aspects, functions and structures in the human body.

Air: It is responsible for all the movements including expansion, contraction, vibration, suppression and elevation etc.

Fire: It is responsible for Hunger, Thirst, Sleep, Vision or Power of eyes and Skin Complexion.

Water: It forms Saliva, blood, urine, sweat, semen and so on.

Earth: It forms Solid structures such as Bones, teeth, nails, muscles, skin, hairs, tissues etc. This element gives strength and forms a solid structure and provides good support to the body.

Space/Ether: It is the subtlest of all the elements and is present in the hollow cavities of the body in the form of Radio Frequencies, Cosmic Rays and star dust, it is also said to be present in the form of Ether, which is basically tiniest level, form of water etc. It is the most unique form from all the above and known forms, so it is also called as 'God Particle' and is present everywhere.

The Vital Life Force/ Energy Flow, also known as 'Prana' in the Human body is directly connected to the 5 elements.

These elements need to be Balanced and this balance should be maintained with constant efforts to achieve the Best Level of Health in the Highest Divine Order.

Etheric Body: The Etheric body is the subtlest body amongst other types. We may call it neutral body. It connects with the higher bodies especially Mental and Emotional. It exchanges, send or receive either positive or negative energy depending up on multiple factors like surroundings, energy fields, status of other bodies with which it is connected. It is also connected with nature, universe and other energy beings who have similar or different electromagnetic field. So basically, etheric body's major and most important function is to make connection/connections (possibly multiple at times) irrespective of positive or negative, high or low frequencies, intra or inter body/electromagnetic fields, type of frequencies, irrespective of time, timeline, space, dimensions and so on.

A person or rather a Personality of the person is a term that actually describes the overall qualities including visibility, functionality, mechanics (Related to Physical Body – Strength, stamina/endurance, flexibility and more all exists parallelly), intelligence (Related to Mental/Psychological Body - thoughts, ideas, creativity and more all exists parallelly), nature (Related to Emotional Body – Happiness, Sadness, Anger, Fear), Belief and Wisdom (Related to Spiritual Body), base

(Related to the 5 Elements' body Present inside our body and as well as in the Nature), Connection (Related to Etheric Body which is also a mean of connection between each and every single thing present in the universe including the human bodies).

Character is an important aspect of personality and which is a very complex combination of Mental/Psychological, Emotional and Spiritual Bodies.

As we have seen so far, everything is interlinked and interconnected and can affect each other that means reaction to every action. And most important fact about the person or personality is that all these characteristics are present at the exact same time parallelly and there could be possible changes in every aspect as per situation, place and timeline, considering the action and reaction law.

And this is what exactly the Quantum Physics is all about. If we understand the quantum reality thoroughly. We can easily understand the same reality about human beings, they are present in all forms (as we know Physical body, Mental Body, Emotional Body, Spiritual Body and Etheric Body in general). These forms could be revealed or explored as per different timelines or as per awakening or consciousness at different levels and these levels or the dimensions of consciousness are possibly achievable by Humans, depending upon Multiple factors. We exist in different realities at the same time, so we need to achieve a great balance in between these.

Do not be slave of any type of the bodies which are present in our quantum reality. Always be the master and control all the bodies, by balancing every aspect of every single body and their different aspects which exist in past, present and future parallelly, so we need to have a great balance in between all these bodies as well as the multiple characteristics of individual bodies in quantum reality and this act of balancing will help us to timely update and upgrade ourselves to higher realms, higher frequencies, higher dimensions with higher awareness, awakening and higher consciousness and overcome darkness and see the true Light, also it will lead us to be, quantum fit. On the contrary part, if we fail to balance these bodies or their individual characteristics this may lead to attract negative frequencies and lead to degradation and destruction of self and resonate into lower dimensions with negative frequencies and vibrations and see no light and fall into dark.

Wake up and be ready. Prepare yourself to start with the right things. Be Aware of the things which may affect your fitness journey. Do research, understand things. Work on self and surroundings. Have great Balance in everything. Attract Positive vibes. Attract light. Be a Light being. Explore Higher Dimensions and Rise to higher realms. Make effective connections. Make new connections with nature and universe. Increase levels of consciousness.

Be Wise Be Fit at quantum levels.

The '4S' Formula

The 4 'S' Formula is, to Start and make your fitness journey successful.

By the way there is a 5th 'S' which stands for 'Success'. And to achieve the 5th 'S', we need to follow the 4 'S' formula.

And what I mean to tell by this 5th 'S' of 'Success' is that, you need to start with right choices and then with constant efforts make progress. You need to analyse and with proper understandings decide and set the actual limit for yourself that how far you want to progress by applying practical and logical thinking. Success could be different for different people at different stages of their fitness journey depending upon different situations, conditions and multiple factors.

But from my point of view the real meaning of Success is 'Maintenance'.

This fitness journey should be sustainable for every single one of you who dare to start it and dream to achieve the greatest success in it. And the actual greatness of the success remains in the sustainability or maintenance of the fitness routine for life time, by fighting with all the obstacles may possibly come in between your fitness journey. The real success lies within keep going, no matter what.

Along with the maintenance or continuity the other important factor is 'Effect' what effect you got by the routine you have been following. If the effect is positive then, know that you are on the right track, but if the effect is negative and it is becoming an obstacle or hurdle in the maintenance of your fitness journey, then it's high time to change your approach, revaluate your choices, chose wisely and utilise your energy, time and money in right direction and stop looking for higher results or higher progress every single time and focus on a safe and effective maintenance which will create a positive impact for lifetime. And by the way Progress and growth are the by-products of the process through which we go in our fitness journey. Or it will happen by default, growth and progress are the part of the process and this journey. So, don't chase them desperately and blindly until you fall down into a deep valley of inconsistency and stuck into the dirt of laziness and depression. And also, don't wait for the things to happen by themselves, act now and take a leap of faith towards your 5th 'S' – 'Success'.

And I guess there must be very few people who achieve this, 'real' success of 'maintenance' with score of 100%.

Let me tell you, I have been working at different levels and in each level of work taught me so much and made me capable to help my people. With my experience of almost 2 decades in the field of Fitness, working with different people with different approaches as a Personal Trainer, as a Coach, as a Mentor, as a Guide, as a teacher and most importantly as an Empathetic and Compassionate Friend and with all my heart, deepest understanding about my work (which includes the knowledge and experience consisting different factors and aspects like technical, theoretical, scientific, practical, psychological, philosophical, logical, judgemental, sensible, experimental, personal and so on) I have found out a great formula to be successful in most of the aspects of life, especially Fitness, Health and wellness.

Follow my 4 'S' formula, never look back or never look for something else or never be confused again about your choices.

1st 'S' Stands 'Safe':

Understand and know what is 'Safe' for you.

As this 'S' is really very important, you need to have a great understanding about your own self. Before starting any routine or before starting your fitness journey, you need to analyse things about yourself, like the type of exercises including in the routine, your body type, current body conditioning, medical or health condition (if any), age, gender and few other important factors or aspects including in your lifestyle as well as workstyle. In terms what suits you or what doesn't suit you or what could be risky for you. You need to gauge and guess the risk factors (Hidden risk factors as well) and also you need to understand the intensity of the risk and what possibly worst impact it could create in your life and with immediate effect or long-term effect, could possibly in near future or in the long run. In some cases, the risk factors may lead to lifelong adverse effect or fatality in the worst scenario. Make sure you are always following safety protocols before even thinking of starting your workouts. Be safe always.

2nd 'S' Stands for 'Simple':

Why Simple?

As I always mention, every aspect of fitness is interlinked and dependent on each other, and parallelly exists.

The first reason behind, keeping your exercises simple is that, simple exercises are always safe. There are least risk factors involved in Simple exercises.

The second reason to select simple exercises is that, Simple exercises are easy to learn, easy to perform and easy to progress and gain perfection with constant efforts. People generally grasp the movements and methods of doing these simple exercises very easily and much faster. Mind muscles coordination becomes effective and the muscle memory remains intact for years, even if you try to perform these simple exercises after a long gap.

Third reason is Simple exercises never become very stressful or too risky if overdone, in-fact they will be beneficial by utilising the percentage of target muscles at it's max in long run. Simple exercises are sustainable, you can do it for years without any risk factors. The person who ever is going to the exercises whether it is a male, female or whether the routine is for children or adults or elderly people or any person with injuries or health issues or specific medical conditions or any kind of physical limitations can do the routine easily, with safety.

So, to make your workouts more effective, to progress early in your workouts and to make them sustainable the selection or choice of exercises should always be 'Simple'.

3rd 'S' stands for 'Suitable':

What is 'Suitable' for you? and How can we make the program customised and suitable depending multiple aspects and factors.

The Suitability means what kind of routine or list of exercises or workout is actually suits you, depending up on multiple factors like age, gender, workstyle, lifestyle, current fitness level and current body conditioning, medical or health condition or injuries (if any), past exercises history or experience, facility or props or equipment available to perform exercises, availability of time, expectations from this exercise routine and so on. By analysing the above-mentioned factors, we can customise the workout plan and make it more suitable for you.

As you must have noticed that, I have not mentioned the 'Fitness Goal' (Short term and long term) purposefully. Also, not mentioned Favourite workouts and the workouts which you dislike the most. Reason behind this is, Long Term Fitness Goal is always like a Big Dream or Fiction, which may or may not come true. But, this Big Dream may come true if you perform and put efforts with hard work and discipline and consistently without any expectations and doing it with the only intension that you are doing it for your own health and your own self.

And to its opposite side, you may not be able to achieve this Big dream ever, reason behind could be your impatience, lack of discipline, short cuts, too much expectations that may lead to disappointment, depression and further lead to discontinuation from the exercise routine, being over enthusiastic, over confidence, overdoing, getting bored thinking that the routine is monotonous and the same, lose confidence, giving up easily, getting under influenced by people or challenges or do it for showing off or egoistic mentality or do it as a competition with others, comparison, overthinking about other people's perception towards you, false beliefs or false proud and ego or doing very intense workouts beyond your capacity without recruiting target muscles or group of muscles to its fullest capacity along with great mind muscle coordination or improper form and postures, doing fancy workouts or aesthetic structural movements or workouts without learning and understanding it in depth, landing up with sport injuries due to inappropriate form or intensity or workouts as per your current fitness level and body conditioning and taking these sports injuries lightly and repeating the past mistakes again and so on.

Now let's discuss about the 'Short term Goal' that means what all things we need to attend in the beginning. What we are supposed to start with in the initial phase and that completely depends up on the Current Fitness Level and internal body conditioning which includes the strength of internal joints, ligaments, tendons or minor internal muscles or deep muscles, core muscle group, flexibility of individual muscles, tendons, ligaments and overall mobility (Range of Motion) of the joints, Negative Structural Changes (Change in the structure of Joints Specifically due to weak/strong opposite muscles), postural changes happened due to imbalance in the muscles due to weakness in the muscles and the main reason for this is lack of conditioning which includes mobility, flexibility, strength and range of motion of the muscles. The negative changes may also happen due to workstyle, sitting posture or sleeping posture or lack of exercise or due to any impact or injury in an accident and few more reasons and possibilities. So 'Short Term Goals' are always decided after the case study. And it could be different for different people. So always take advice from an expert in the field.

4th 'S' stands for 'Sustainable':

How can we make our workouts 'Sustainable'?

This is very important factor from the point of view of one's consistency in the workout routine and progress in it.

Many people start their fitness routine with a great excitement. They are very enthusiastic and are very sincere and particular about it. Many are very dedicated in the beginning phase. They keep too many expectations right from the first day itself. Most of them are very confident about it and some are over confident too. They think they can do anything, they also think they can do many things at the same time and most of them wish to do multiple things like Running, Yoga,

Functional Training, Power Yoga, Spinning, Heavy Weight Training or even power lifting in that matter. But most of them miserably fail because of few reasons mentioned below:

- Setting Unrealistic Goals.
- Over Expectations.
- Impatience.
- Trying different options right from the beginning.
- Won't give sufficient amount of time for recovery.
- Over exertion.
- Disappointment on not achieving quick results.
- Lack of Discipline.
- Lack of motivation.
- Always blame your surroundings or people for your inconsistency.
- No accountability.
- Negative Approach.
- Depression.
- Mood swings due to imbalanced hormones.
- Stress due to work or family issues or even stressing out because of not able to maintain the workout routine or unable to take out time for your workouts.

- ❖ Laziness.
- ❖ Trust issues, about self or on the people who help in your fitness journey.
- ❖ Too many Doubts or unclear mind.
- ❖ Tiredness.
- ❖ Doing the same routine and the same workouts becoming monotonous or boring.
- ❖ Lack of time.
- ❖ Due to work.
- ❖ Egoistic approach.
- ❖ Comparison.
- ❖ Repeating the same mistakes again and again.
- ❖ Having false impression about the progress or results.
- ❖ Competition.
- ❖ Ignoring bodily signals and continuing with same or higher intensity.
- ❖ Ignoring body/muscle/joint pain.
- ❖ Ignoring or underestimating the process of recovery.
- ❖ Aiming for higher intensity in every single workout.
- ❖ Pushing too hard, too long and every time they workout.

- ❖ No fact checking or researching, before starting anything new.
- ❖ Starting with unsuitable or wrong workout program without any customization in it.
- ❖ Extending workouts for long period of time with higher intensities.
- ❖ Imbalance in everything.
- ❖ Underestimate simple and easy things which could be beneficial and safe.
- ❖ Focus on just one or two things and ignoring other important factors.
- ❖ No preplanning or following the things randomly.
- ❖ Following anything or anyone blindly.
- ❖ Being Over aggressive - Over aggression may lead to accidents.
- ❖ Busy schedule.
- ❖ Illness.
- ❖ Sports injury.
- ❖ Dependency, either on Coach/Trainer or a gym buddy/friend/partner or location or equipment used etc.

Such and many more reasons possibly could hamper your consistency in the workouts and by default affect the sustainability of the workout routine.

Solutions:

For every problem you need to have right solutions and options available to make your fitness journey unstoppable and make your workout routine more sustainable.

Here are few solutions for the problems due to which your workout routine gets affected and you are not able to Start, Restart or Maintain your Fitness Journey.

- ❖ Always do current assessment of your own health and fitness levels.
- ❖ Focus on conditioning.
- ❖ Always start with the basics and most simple workouts, exercises, yogic poses, stretches and movements.
- ❖ Keep lots of patience for everything
- ❖ Have faith and trust yourself, on the plan, on the process and on your fitness journey.
- ❖ Have Clarity of thoughts about the thing which you have, about the things which are in your control and about the things which are not in your control.
- ❖ Understand your own self, current conditions and present situations and act accordingly.
- ❖ Always have a positive approach about every possible thing in the process.

- Do not complicate things.
- Chose safe and wise options which suits you practically and logically.
- Take advice from experts.
- Do your own research.
- Do not go for extreme levels for anything.
- Do not follow anything or anyone blindly.
- Do not compare with others.
- Have an egoless approach always.
- Do not follow anything randomly.
- Get a good and suitable workout plan customised for yourself from a fitness expert.
- Keep Track record.
- Have a clarity of thoughts about Results or the process of progress with a sensible, practical, logical, wise and positive approach.
- Keep calm in every situation.
- Do not be over aggressive.
- Always have balance in everything.
- Do not focus on only one or two things.
- Do not ignore important factors.
- Always check for facts and research.
- Learn from mistakes and Repeat no Mistakes.
- Avoid overdoing.

- ❖ Understand the signals of the body, mind and gut feelings.
- ❖ Progress happens Naturally and by default if the body receives right nutrition and recovers full, even though it is less or comparatively slow but, it is a good progress.
- ❖ Always prefer safety over fast progress and short cuts.
- ❖ Do not get over whelmed with progress.
- ❖ Do not keep short term goals and do not stop once you achieve the short-term goals.

Whatever you do need to be balanced. It needs to be in your control. And in case of any exercise, workout or treatment you are undertaking should always be pain free. Then only, you will be able to make your fitness journey sustainable. And also see the desired changes in yourselves at quantum levels.

Break the Ice

Talk to someone about your thoughts on your body image or weight or talk about your fitness levels. Express your desire of starting the fitness journey. Do not hesitate to connect with an expert, who can guide you throughout your fitness journey. It will be a learning phase for you, because you will be learning many things which you were not aware of in the past from the experts. And most importantly you receive the knowledge and it is never a waste. Knowledge is power. Knowledge is for Life. So, learn it, earn it and apply it and experience the change in your life. Find a Genuine, Experienced, Knowledgeable and Wise Fitness Expert, who will have the right understanding of your Body's Physical, physiological and Psychological State. Explain the problems you are facing, explain your Current Condition in terms of Health and Fitness, express your thoughts about your expectations, Tell your past or history about your Health as well as Fitness or Exercise routines. Explain the situations or reasons why you were not able to stick to any routine so far or why you had to stop it. Your current occupation, mental status, family background, stress levels, medical condition, answer all the questions asked by your Fitness Expert. If you feel that anything related or not related to your health and fitness but you feel it might be helpful or just for your satisfaction, feel free to add. And accordingly, He/ She will be able to Create a 'Blue Print' of your 'Fitness Journey'.

Mindset or psychology plays very important role in fitness.

So, in your fitness journey always have clarity of thought about the thing you are doing, why are you doing and where these things are going to lead you in future. Once your mind is crystal clear and good to go, then start with a great positive approach and never doubt on your decision and never ever look back, just keep going to achieve your aim.

Benefits of Exercise

Exercise has many physical, mental and emotional benefits. Here are some of the most significant benefits of regular exercise:

1. **Physical Health:** Regular exercise can improve physical health by reducing the risk of chronic diseases such as heart disease, stroke, diabetes, and some types of cancer. It can also lower blood pressure, improve cholesterol levels, and strengthen bones and muscles.

2. **Mental Health:** Exercise has been shown to improve mood and reduce symptoms of anxiety and depression. It also increases the release of endorphins, which are natural chemicals in the brain that improve mood and reduce stress.

3. **Weight Management:** Exercise is an important component of a weight management program. It can help you burn calories, increase muscle mass, and boost metabolism.

4. **Better Sleep:** Exercise has been shown to improve sleep quality and help people fall asleep faster.

5. **Increased Energy:** Regular exercise can boost energy levels and improve overall physical and mental performance.

6. **Improved Brain Function:** Exercise has been shown to improve cognitive function, memory, and concentration.
7. **Increased Confidence:** Regular exercise can help boost self-esteem and increase feelings of confidence.
8. **Social Connection:** Exercise can also provide opportunities for social interaction and can help to improve relationships and build a sense of community.

Exercise is a crucial aspect of maintaining a healthy and balanced lifestyle, and the benefits are numerous and far-reaching.

Observe and analyse the effects of workouts:

The effects of a workout and exercise routine can be significant and wide-ranging. Here are some of the ways in which regular exercise can benefit the body and mind:

Physical health benefits:

- **Improved cardiovascular health:** Regular exercise can help improve heart health by lowering blood pressure, increasing heart strength, and reducing the risk of heart disease.
- **Stronger muscles and bones:** Exercise, especially weight-bearing activities, can help

build and maintain strong muscles and bones, reducing the risk of osteoporosis and other bone diseases.

- **Better weight management:** Regular exercise can help you maintain a healthy weight by burning calories and reducing the risk of obesity.
- **Improved flexibility and balance:** Exercise can help improve flexibility and balance, reducing the risk of falls and other accidents.
- **Better sleep:** Exercise has been shown to improve sleep quality, helping you feel more rested and refreshed during the day.

Mental health benefits:

- **Reduced stress and anxiety:** Exercise has been shown to help reduce stress and anxiety levels by releasing endorphins and other mood-enhancing chemicals.
- **Improved mood:** Regular exercise has been linked to improved mood and a reduced risk of depression.
- **Enhanced cognitive function:** Exercise has been shown to improve cognitive function and reduce the risk of age-related decline in brain function.

- **Increased self-esteem and confidence:** Regular exercise can help increase self-esteem and confidence by improving physical appearance and fitness levels.

It's important to note that the benefits of exercise can vary greatly depending on the type and intensity of the exercise, as well as the individual's age, health, and fitness level. It's always best to consult with a healthcare professional before starting a new exercise routine to determine what's best for you.

Regular exercise has also been linked to several other positive health outcomes, such as:

- **Improved immune system function:** Exercise has been shown to improve the body's immune system function, helping to fight off illnesses and infections.
- **Improved digestion:** Exercise can help stimulate the digestive system, improving digestion and reducing the risk of digestive disorders.
- **Reduced risk of chronic diseases:** Regular exercise has been linked to a reduced risk of several chronic diseases, including type 2 diabetes, certain types of cancer, and Alzheimer's disease.

- **Improved sexual function:** Exercise has been shown to improve sexual function and increase sexual desire in both men and women.
- **Increased energy levels:** Regular exercise has been shown to increase energy levels, allowing you to be more active and productive throughout the day.

The effects of exercise can be seen not only in physical health, but also in other areas of life. For example, exercise has been shown to improve academic performance in children, increase productivity in the workplace, and enhance overall quality of life. Regular exercise and a well-rounded workout routine can have a profound impact on both physical and mental health, and can lead to a wide range of positive outcomes. Whether you're looking to improve your physical fitness, boost your mood, or simply lead a healthier lifestyle, exercise can be a valuable tool for achieving your goals.

Greater State of Physical Health:

This includes a variety of factors, such as:

1. **Adequate nutrition:** Consuming a balanced and nutritious diet that provides the body with the necessary vitamins, minerals, and macronutrients to function optimally.

2. **Regular physical activity:** Engaging in regular exercise and physical activity that helps maintain a healthy weight, improves cardiovascular health, and strengthens bones and muscles.
3. **Optimal sleep:** Getting enough quality sleep, which is essential for physical and mental recovery, memory consolidation, and overall health.
4. **Chronic disease management:** Managing any chronic conditions, such as diabetes, hypertension, or heart disease, through proper treatment, medication, and lifestyle modifications.
5. **Avoidance of harmful substances:** Abstaining from harmful substances, such as tobacco, alcohol, and drugs, which can have negative impacts on physical health.
6. **Stress management:** Managing stress levels through techniques such as mindfulness, exercise, and relaxation. Chronic stress can have negative effects on physical health, including increasing the risk of heart disease and weakening the immune system.
7. **Hydration:** Drinking enough water to maintain proper hydration levels, which is important for many physiological processes, including

regulating body temperature and removing waste products.

8. **Preventive health screenings:** Undergoing preventive health screenings, such as regular check-ups and screenings for cancers and other chronic diseases, to detect any potential health problems early and receive prompt treatment.

9. **Healthy relationships:** Building and maintaining healthy relationships with friends, family, and loved ones, which can have positive effects on mental and emotional health, and in turn, physical health.

10. **Positive outlook:** Cultivating a positive outlook and maintaining a healthy mental state, which can boost immunity, reduce stress, and improve overall health.

Achieving a greater state of physical health requires making positive lifestyle choices, engaging in regular physical activity, and seeking proper medical care when necessary. By taking these steps, individuals can improve their physical well-being and reduce the risk of chronic diseases. Physical health is not a static condition, but rather a journey that requires continuous effort and attention. By making positive lifestyle choices, engaging in regular physical activity, and seeking proper medical care, when necessary, individuals can improve their physical well-being and achieve a greater state of physical health.

Greater State of Mental Health:

Having good mental health is essential for overall health and well-being, and can greatly impact an individual's quality of life. It is important to note that mental health is not just the absence of mental illness, but rather a state of dynamic balance and resilience that allows individuals to flourish and thrive.

A person in a greater state of mental health may also have the following qualities:

1. **Positive Thinking:** They have a positive outlook on life, look for the good in situations, and have a healthy perspective on challenges and failures.
2. **Emotional Stability:** They are able to regulate their emotions and maintain a stable mood, even in stressful or challenging situations.
3. **Good Self-Care:** They engage in activities that promote physical, emotional and mental well-being, such as exercise, healthy eating, and self-reflection.
4. **Strong Support System:** They have a network of supportive friends and family members who provide emotional and practical support.

5. **Adaptability:** They are able to adjust to change, uncertainty and new situations in a positive and resilient way.
6. **Empathy:** They have the ability to understand and connect with others, and show compassion and kindness towards others.
7. **Sense of Purpose:** They have a clear sense of purpose and meaning in life, and are motivated to pursue their goals and aspirations.

It's important to note that mental health is a dynamic and ongoing process, and everyone experiences ups and downs in their mental well-being. The key is to develop and maintain habits and practices that promote and sustain a greater state of mental health.

Maintaining a greater state of mental health requires a proactive approach and a commitment to self-care. Here are some steps you can take to improve your mental health:

1. **Practice good self-care habits:** Get enough sleep, exercise regularly, eat a healthy diet, and engage in activities that bring you joy and relaxation.
2. **Connect with others:** Build strong relationships with friends and family, join a community group or organization, and consider therapy or counselling if needed.

3. **Manage stress:** Learn effective stress management techniques such as mindfulness, meditation, deep breathing, and exercise.
4. **Cultivate positive thinking:** Practice gratitude, positive self-talk, and focus on the present moment.
5. **Take care of your physical health:** Regular exercise, healthy eating, and getting enough sleep can all have a positive impact on mental health.
6. **Seek professional help:** If you're struggling with symptoms of depression, anxiety, or any other mental health issue, consider seeking help from a mental health professional.
7. **Set achievable goals:** Having a clear sense of purpose and a plan for achieving your goals can provide a sense of direction and meaning in life.

Remember, good mental health is not just about avoiding mental health problems, but about actively pursuing and maintaining a greater state of well-being. By taking care of yourself and seeking support when needed, you can cultivate a greater state of mental health and enjoy a higher quality of life.

Body Weight and Confusion

There has been an observation always, that many people are obsessed about their body weight. And the same, people are always confused about it. To get rid of this confusion, we should properly understand and have clarity of thoughts, about our body weight. Once we know how our body functions, what it is made up of and why the weight is changing or remaining constant, then it becomes very easy to start your fitness journey with complete positive thoughts and a crystal-clear Mind.

The Human Body Weight:

Human Body weight can be defined as the weight or mass of a person, without any item located on it. And is can be measured in units like LBS or Pounds or Kilograms.

The Human Body Weight is consisting of the following things:

Before knowing this, we need to understand the human body, what exactly it is, and how it functions. Human body is very complex and it's not fixed like a machine or it doesn't remain constant all the time. There are lot many things that are going on, right from inside. There are many systems inside the human body, these systems are functioned or run under different organs and most of the systems and functions are interlinked with each other in some or the other way. But all the systems, functions and organs are directly related to Human brain. Brain controls all the Functions and Systems.

There are many functions and works which are carried out, inside the human body even while a person is into deep sleep. There are lot many changes take place inside the human body which usually we don't come to know from outside on a daily basis or over the period of time.

Let's understand the Gross structure of the human body and the different categories fall under the body weight:

1) Bones:

There is a gross structure of bones which includes the major parts like, The Skull, The Spinal Column, The Rib cage, The Limbs (Upper Extremity/Body), The Pelvic joint, The Limbs (Lower Extremity/Body), etc.

This is the most basic foundation and structure of a Human Body. And the weight of bones all together is approximately 14% of the total body weight.

2) Internal Organs:

The weight of different major organs which runs different systems and functions. Here is the list of internal organs:

The Brain, The Heart, The Lungs, The Liver, The Bladder, The Kidneys, The Stomach, The Intestine etc.

Apart from these major Internal Organs there are different glands attached to different major organs, veins, arteries and so on, including these there are total 78 Organs. The list is huge. And the weight of the organs all together and on an individual organ basis may differ from person to person, depending up on person's Age, Gender, Race, Genetics, Location and so on.

3) Body Water:

This is also an important part, all type of fluids and liquids which consists of:

Water, Chemicals, Hormones, Mucus, Saliva, Liquids, Fluids, Blood, Acids, Alkali, Toxic wastes like Urine and so on.

In total, there are 26 Fluids in the body. At different locations and some are present and in constant function all the time, but some are secreted or released or created by some particular actions for example Tears are related with emotions, Sweats is released if we do physical exercises or if we are in hot and humid climates. It's the natural mechanism of body.

The quantity and weight of these fluids may be different from person to person or as per the external factors like environment or as per the internal factors like body mechanism in the functioning of different systems and it's not same every time for the same person as well.

So, the total Water inside the body in different forms, including all sub categories, is on an average of 60% to 67% in adult Men, but comparatively it is slightly less in Women and i.e., 52% to 55% of the Total Body Weight. That means, Body water covers a larger area and it's very important for the proper functioning of Human Body.

4) Skin:

Skin is the largest organ in the human body, that's why it is counted separately. Skin is the outer covering of the body and it has 7 layers of ectodermal tissues. And it guards the underlying muscle tissues, ligaments, bones and internal organs. Human skin weighs around 3Kg to 4Kg on an average, and it may vary person to person, depending upon Height, Genetical Structure and quality of the skin layers (Thickness) and so on.

5) Muscles:

A Muscle can be defined as a Group of tissues which have the ability to contract together, depending up on the type –

1) Voluntarily to generate force against resistance after receiving signals from the brain (Controlled by CNS) i.e., called Voluntary or Skeletal Muscles.

2) Contract slowly and rhythmically, to contribute in the constant or timely functioning of any organ and it's an involuntary repeated movement, Controlled by ANS (Autonomic Nervous System).

3) The Muscle contractions here are Involuntary, Rhythmic but strong. Constant functioning under the control of ANS and are called as Cardiac Muscles.

We have taken information about the Organs in one of the previous points, so smooth Muscle and cardiac muscles both types are covered, under the section of Organs. So, we have considered the weight of these 2 types of muscles already.

Here we will majorly consider the Skeletal Muscles. And the average percentage of the Muscles in Men and Women, majorly depends on the age.

Here are some rough figures.

On an Average, Normal ranges for **muscle mass** are:

Ages 20-39: **75-89** percent for **men**, **63-75.5** percent for **women**. Ages 40-59: **73-86** percent for men, **62-73.5** percent for **women**.

6) Body Fat:

There are 6 types of body fat:

1) Essential Fat:

This fat is essential for a good health. It helps in regulating body temperature, helps in Vitamin absorption and also helps in the production of fertility hormones. Essential Fat is not very visible, but it's present all over the body. Essential Fat is considered very Good for the body. And it shouldn't be targeted for the fat loss.

In females essential Fat generally ranges in between 8% to 12% for a good health. And for Men, the ideal range of essential Fat is 3% to 5% for a good health, of total body weight.

7) **Brown Fat:**

Brown Fat is Considered as a 'Good' Fat. The main function of Brown Fat is to Burn Energy. And it also maintains the body's Core temperature. Brown Fat doesn't get stored and it's easy to burn. Especially it's good to have brown Fat in Cooler climates to maintain body's Core temperature.

Brown Fat is produced automatically, just by maintaining Essential Fat levels. Essential Fat is a great support system for brown Fat.

8) **White Fat:**

White fat can be considered as Neutral, but as per the situation it may act good or bad.

White fat is body's largest energy storage system. It produces adiponectin, so it's essential for the management of insulin and to maintain a healthy blood sugar balance. It also produces leptin and it manages hunger. It is also involved in the production of growth hormone and cortisol. There are so many important works for white fat, but it can be bad if it is present in a large quantity. In greater quantity, white fat can cause insulin resistance and raise the risk of weight gain and further it may lead to serious health concerns.

Stubborn excess fat on thighs, hips and abdomen are the signs of higher white fat levels. A regular exercise routine with right kind of exercises, help to reduce white fat levels over the period of time. Also controlled portion meals, may promote the transition of white fat to Brown Fat.

9) Beige Fat:

Beige fat is considered as a good fat. Beige fat is created when the body is exposed to stress, leading to change the colour of white fat to 'Beige'. While a high level of beige fat isn't really a target goal, it's definitely a step in the right direction to maintain healthy levels of good brown Fat, it essentially allows for the transformation and burning of bad fat as thermal energy to maintain body's Core temperature.

The beige fat's role in transforming white fat to useful thermal energy makes it a good target for weight loss. Exercise can create a good physical stress for transforming white fat to beige fat due to the production of the hormone irisin. The key here is stress, so aim for at least 75 Minutes vigorous exercise each week. But make sure that, you should always start with less time duration as a beginner and with consistency, the desired time duration can be achieved.

5) **Subcutaneous Fat:**

Subcutaneous Fat can be considered as Neutral same like white Fat. Subcutaneous Fat is present just under the skin. It accounts for approximately 90% of overall body fat percentage. Commonly accumulating as Stubborn Thigh Fat in females or around the abdomen in Males. Subcutaneous Fat is responsible for the sex hormone estrogen. Because estrogen plays a larger role in female fertility, females tend to have higher levels of subcutaneous fat. This fat also acts as a cushion between Muscle and skin tissue for protection and comfort.

Subcutaneous Fat is essential but too much, particularly around the abdomen increase the risk and health complications. Because body stores subcutaneous fat as an emergency backup in case of starvation or caloric deprivation, this type of fat is hardest to target. A reduction in calories consumed, a focus on improved nutrition to avoid refined carbs and processed foods, and regular high intensity exercise can over the period of time, burn off excess subcutaneous fat.

6) **Visceral fat:**

Visceral fat is a bad fat. It is present in the abdominal cavity, present in between the organs. It accumulates and secrets retinol-binding protein 4, a known culprit in insulin resistance higher levels of visceral fat is also linked to an increased risk of colorectal and breast Cancer, dementia, stroke and Alzheimer's disease. Visceral fat levels generally increase with age.

One of the best ways to decrease visceral fat levels is to focus on diet. Avoid processed foods. Increase intake of lean protein, unsaturated fatty foods, whole grains and fibre. Improve the sleeping patterns, with 7 to 9 hours sleep is beneficial. Abdominal strength training plus targeting bigger muscles like lower body muscles exercises will increase caloric burn and help to reduce overall fat percentage.

BMI (Body Mass Index):

Body mass index is a value derived from the mass and height of a person. The BMI is defined as the body mass divided by the square of the body height, and is expressed in units of kg/m^2, resulting from mass in kilograms and height in metres.

Every Hight has an ideal body weight range, so it will be different for different people.

Commonly Known Categories of Weight:

1) **Underweight:** Basically, these people fall under the category of 'Ectomorph'. If your **BMI** is less than 18.5, it falls within the **underweight range**.

2) **Ideal/ Normal Weight:** People having their body weight in the normal range fall under the category called 'Mesomorph'. If your **BMI** is 18.5 to 24.9, it falls within the normal or Healthy Weight **range**.

3) **Over Weight:** People with more body weight than the normal range, fall under 'Endomorph' Category. If your **BMI** is 25.0 to 29.9, it falls within the **overweight range**.

4) **Obese:** Obesity is the next level of overweight category, but it still falls under the category of 'Endomorph' body type. Only the risk factor increases further because of more fat.

Obesity is a complex disease involving an excessive amount of body fat. **Obesity** isn't just a cosmetic concern. It is a medical problem that increases your risk of other diseases and health problems, such as heart disease, diabetes, high blood pressure and certain cancers.

Obesity often results from taking in more calories than are burned by exercise and normal daily activities.

Obesity occurs when a person's body mass index is 25 to 29.9 or greater (Depending on different factors). The excessive body fat increases the risk of serious health problems.

Obesity Levels: These are the average ranges.

There are 3 levels of obesity, with every increased level, the risk factor increases.

Obesity Class 1 - BMI = 30 to 34.9 – High Risk Factors.

Obesity Class 2 – BMI = 35 to 39.9 – Very High-Risk Factors.

Obesity Class 3 – BMI 40 or higher – Highest-Risk Factors involved.

Symptoms of Obesity:

Frequent Symptoms for Adults:

Symptoms of obesity can negatively impact one's daily life. For adults, frequent symptoms include:

Excess body fat accumulation (particularly around the waist)

Shortness of breath.

Sweating (more than usual)

Snoring

Trouble sleeping

Skin problems (from moisture accumulating in the folds of skin)

Inability to perform simple physical tasks (that one could easily perform before weight gain)

Fatigue (from mild to extreme)

Pain (commonly in the back and joints)

Psychological impact (negative self-esteem, depression, shame, social isolation)

Frequent Symptoms for Children and Adolescents:

Eating disorders

Fatty tissue deposits (may be noticeable in the breast area)

The appearance of stretch marks on the hips and back

Dark velvety skin around the neck and other areas.

Shortness of breath with physical activity

Insomnia

Constipation.

G I reflux

Poor self-esteem

Early puberty in girls/delayed puberty in boys

Orthopaedic problems (such as flat feet or dislocated hips OR any other structural defect caused because of obesity over the period of time.)

Risk Factors:

High blood pressure (hypertension) or heart disease from the heart working hard to pump blood to more surface area of the body

High Cholesterol levels (fatty deposits that can block arteries) leading to stroke, heart attack and other complications

Stroke (from high cholesterol levels and high blood pressure)

Type 2 diabetes (nearly 50% of type 2 diabetes cases are directly linked to obesity)

Some types of cancers.

Asthma

Kidney Diseases, can occur from chronic high blood pressure, that damages the kidneys.

Osteoarthritis from excess weight causing an additional strain on the joints, bones, and muscles.

Gallbladder Diseases.

Sleep apnoea, as fat deposits in the neck and tongue block airways.

Gastroesophageal Reflux, Hiatal Hernia, and Heartburn caused by excess weight pushing on the valve at the top of the stomach. This allows stomach acid to leak into the oesophagus.

Note: BMI isn't always an accurate measurement of body fat content.

For example, some athletes are very muscular and because their weight reflects a high level of muscle mass. This may wrongly qualify them for the obesity category, although they have very little body fat.

Similarly, if someone having less fat percentage and good bone density (Heavy Bones) or good quality of bones, on the scale the weight of the person might be at the higher side and so as the BMI. This also will be categorised wrongly into obese category.

There could be multiple examples like this.

So always think wisely about your Fitness, Health and Lifestyle, because what we see isn't always correct or exact the way it is. Check the other side of the coin as well.

Different Factors that affect body weight:

A) The Factors which we cannot change:

Family Background – Our Roots. Our Ancestors. Their Work and Lifestyle. Family Culture. Their Eating habits.

Family History, Heredity, Genes – Height, length and Thickness of bones, Bone density (Very Important Factor), Body Symmetry or body structure, runs in the family (Thickness of Muscles or volume of muscle in specific spots or areas, so as the layer fat, that might be different from others). Each family has a different body structure pattern, which might be identical or different from others.

Race or Ethnicity or Locality and Climate – Mainly there is a difference in the body structure as per the climate and location. A person from America, definitely must be having a different body type and structure than a person from Africa. Similarly, a person who lives in Hills or mountain area, must be having a different body structure who lives in a coastal area.

Body Type:

There are three categories:

Ectomorph – Thin Frame.

Mesomorph – Medium Frame.

Endomorph – Thick Frame.

Age – With the aging process, most of the body's internal systems slows down naturally and that leads to Low BMR (Basal Metabolic Rate) and increased weight (Fat).

Gender or Sex – There is a Hormonal difference in Male and Female body and accordingly there is a difference in Fat percentage. Females have more fat percentage compare to Males.

A) **The Factors which we can change:**

Family Culture and Habits – Many families run a family business, so accordingly there are specific habits or lifestyle or workstyle which everyone follows in the family. Their routine is set. And they follow it for years. But if some habits or the lifestyle or workstyle is not good for health of the family members, then there is always a scope to change it or make necessary corrections.

Environment and Surroundings – In this there are lot of things we can consider, the work place, residence place, locality and culture. Availability of local and seasonal foods.

Eating Habits – Eating Junk Food, Packaged Foods, Bakery Products, too oily, Too Sweet, Too Spicy, Overeating, Wrong timings of meals, Frequent Fasting,

Following Crash Diets or Fad Diets. Having foods which have artificial sweeteners, colours, taste enhancers in it. Drinking Aerated cold drinks very often. These eating habits may lead to increased weight.

Physical Activity – Lack of Physical activity Or Exercise is the major reason to put on the weight and Fat.

Workstyle – If you have a Desk job or Sedentary work, the chances to increase weight and fat are far more.

Hormonal Imbalance:

Thyroid (Hypothyroidism and Hyperthyroidism):

Problems related to thyroid gland and the secretion of thyroid hormone in Under or Over proportion amounts. Which may lead to slow down or increased BMR depending up on the condition. And may further lead to put on more fat or weight loss or muscles loss.

It could be reversal with a lifestyle change, diet, yoga and exercises.

PCOS and PCOD:

Problems related to Menstrual Cycle in Women. Irregularity of the Menstrual Cycle and if more complicated, may lead to infertility.

It could be reversal with a lifestyle change, diet, yoga and exercises.

Sleep Pattern: A good sound sleep for sufficient and required time duration help in good recovery. Lack of sleep is also one of the major reasons for increased body weight.

Another sleep related issue is that, sleeping late and waking up late. This also leads to slow down the internal systems and BMR and leads to increased weight.

Addictions: Alcohol, Cigarettes and other addictions, also interrupt the work and efficiency of internal organs and their workflow and systems. Leads to low BMR. Because of alcohol, more unnecessary calorie intake happens and that puts on more weight and fat.

Medicines: Some medicines might stimulate your appetite. Some medicines might be having some content of steroids. This causes you to eat more and gain extra weight. Some medicines might affect your body's metabolism. This causes your body to burn calories at a slower rate. Some medicines may have content of sedatives and that will lead to deep sleep for more time for fast recovery from ailment.

Water Retention/ Bloating/ Swelling: Bloating occurs due to water retention, which, like many other PMS symptoms, is caused by hormonal changes. **Weight gain** may be associated with other PMS symptoms, such as: water retention, which can slightly **increase** your **weight** ("water **weight**") food cravings that may cause you to overeat or eat unhealthy foods.

To be clear, we're talking about water weight as bloating and not chronic water retention, which indicates a malfunctioning of the kidney or hormones. Bloating is sporadic, usually triggered by diet or lifestyle, and can be remedied without a trip to the doctor -- though the kidneys do play an important role. "The kidney is a dynamic organ,". "It decides whether to hold on to water. If you've had too much salt the night before, then your kidneys will hold on to more water to dilute or correct that salty imbalance... Then they flush it all out."

Individual Psychology / Mental Block: Self-esteem plays a significant role in **weight gain**. If you're already carrying extra pounds, your self-esteem may be low, which triggers an emotional response that sends you back to overeating time and again.

Confusions about the Body Weight:

Constant Fluctuation in the body Weight:

Due to body's natural mechanism, there are lot many changes, which are taking place constantly inside the body. So, the body is never at rest or at a constant/ fixed condition or phase. So, it is obvious that we cannot expect the same weight all the time. There might be fluctuations or difference in the body weight time to time. But it's not a thing to worry about. Just focus on the regime.

The best solution to stop the fluctuation in the weight is to stop checking the weight every now and then, Simple!

Do not check weight very often.

Fixed or No difference in Body Weight for long time:

Body type or Genes

Disciplined lifestyle in term of exercise routine and Nutrition.

No change in weight despite of regular Exercise and Diet:

There might be Multiple reasons like,

Increment in Muscles.

Hormonal Imbalance, especially thyroid.

No increment in weight:

Lack of required Nutrition, Rest and Strength training (In Case, if someone is trying hard to Gain body Weight and Muscles). Body type could be the important factor responsible for this.

Comparison of Weight with others:

Many people compare themselves with others. But that is not right, everyone is of a different make and everyone is living a different life, so we should never compare about the weight or change or difference or results in regards to body weight.

Dependency on Machines and devices and gadgets:

No device in the world gives guarantee of 100 % accuracy. There will be fluctuation always. Human body is way beyond complex structure. There are lot of changes happening in every fraction of second. So, nobody can give assurance that the state of body from inside will remain constant all the time.

Also consider these factors as well, that whether the Machine or Device is functioning well or there is some technical problem in it and it need to be repaired. Or sometimes if the battery of the machine or device is low, then also it might show the fluctuation in the numbers or might show completely different numbers. Or it may show some error. We need to consider all this.

Too Calculative Mindset:

Never be too calculative about your weight or calorie consumption or any other assumed ways like Various Lab Tests, BMI through a Machine or Manually Calculated and so on to evaluate your current health status, because body is very complicated and not constant, a lot many functions are carried out at the same time, so we cannot expect the body to function same way always. Imagine, what if the Machine is not Functioning properly and might give wrong values with slight changes, are we still supposed to believe it? and change our perception and let our thought process be affected because of wrong values in the report papers.

And as we see every day is not same, our thoughts are also not the same, sometimes they are very positive and sometimes they might be negative. As Human psychology is different time to time and cannot remain the same all the time, similarly physiology and physical body will also not remain in the same condition all the time, there is one thing that remains constant and i.e., 'CHANGE'. A 'Slight' change or difference every time we may notice, but it will be there always.

In some situations, **values** might fluctuate **drastically** within minimum time, for example:

When a person catches any **viral infection**, the body condition changes and so as the **values**.

Similarly, when a person takes any kind of **Stimulants,** the body condition will change and so as the **values**.

Pre-Meal - Post meal, Pre-Workout – Post Workouts and so on.

Different conditions – Different Values.

Physical Condition, Physiological Condition or Psychological Condition, everything Matters in Regards to the Evaluative Values of a Person.

Even though the Tests are preferred to do empty stomach or while fasting so that we get accuracy in the values, but it won't show exact the same at different times or days or we may consider the psychological condition of the person at that time.

Which is why, we need to be very clear about one thing, that we should never ever be dependent on the Evaluations or Calculations. We should not get depressed by the values, because they are not permanent and there is always a scope for positive change in the values. So, don't trust anything **Blindly.** Critical thinking is better than, having no thoughts about any situation and accept it. Especially if the situation which is of your concern, you should definitely have clarity of thoughts.

Over Expectations:

Always be wise and have a matured approach towards your Fitness, Health and Lifestyle. So first of all, study and analyse your own body, how it functions as per your current age, lifestyle, workstyle and fitness level. Then chose right options for you. Start with the process with positive approach.

Trust the process. Never hurry, Never Rush. Do not keep any expectations and then receive unexpected. Keep Patience. Accept the reality. Never compare yourself with others. Know that you are doing it for your own self, so never try to do the things to just to show others, or avoid the things which doesn't suite you. Choose a sustainable way. If you are losing your weight very fast, then there might be some problem in the system or the hormones or the techniques used in terms of Nutrition and Exercises might not be the correct. Please check. Do not push yourself very hard, don't be very harsh on your own self. Self-care first and then self-development.

Solutions:

Make your mind clear about certain things. There has to be clarity of thoughts. Keep your Mind positive always and you will be healthy soon and your body weight will be maintained in the ideal weight category always.

Never Consider the Weight, if you are into ideal weight Category. And if you are into underweight or overweight category, consider the weight just for reference. Always Consider the fat percentage, but only when your fitness journey is going on, you are putting constant efforts. And body weight shouldn't be the only criteria to track the results or progress in your fitness journey. But if you haven't started your fitness journey yet, then definitely you should consider your weight.

Take it seriously. And Start with your Fitness Journey now.

A regular exercise routine definitely helps. But Constant efforts with patience without expectations is the only key to Greatest Success.

And yes, there will be fluctuations always in the weight, because even though if we are sitting or sleeping, we feel we are constant, but there are many changes and fluctuations happening because of so many systems are in constant work. Our body is like a whole universe in itself.

So as I mentioned earlier, we have to first understand the weight we carry includes many things like, bone weight, muscle weight, weight of different organs (Heart, Lungs, Liver, Kidneys, Intestine etc etc.), Different Chemicals(Hormones), Water, blood, excretory products, Skin, Hairs, Food we eat, water we drink and Finally the Fat (Certain amount of fat is also necessary, because the fat around our internal organs protects them, fat is also responsible to regulate body temperature and in case of females, it's good to carry little more extra fat while they are pregnant because some type of fats plays important role in the production of hormones etc etc) And Most of us wants to get rid of this excessive fat, we always are mistaken to understand or mix this fat weight with the other essential different weights present in the body.

Do you think if we reduce the weight from the above-mentioned list except Fat, will it be a good idea?

(If the bone weight is reduced, If Muscles or blood is reduced, if internal organs' weight reduced?)

What will happen to us? So please try to understand.

What is more important to us?

1) Weight Loss? Or 2) Fat Loss? And that too which type of fat?

If you still say Weight Loss, then nobody can help you to understand this fact, which you might be denying conveniently.

And if you say 'Fat Loss' then there is a right process for it. And any process takes time.

Also, we need to understand, that while we are in a regular workout routine and if we are following right kind of exercises and providing right nutritional values on daily basis and taking proper rest as well, then there will be increment in Muscle Mass (It's the healthiest way), The quality of bones and Joints will be improved. And because of increased Muscles, you won't see any major difference in your weight, but there must be a difference in Measurements because of increased Metabolic Rate (Ability of the body to burn calories throughout the day and night, without doing any activity or while the body is in the state of Rest. And this is possible, just because of increased Muscle Mass).

And Hypertrophy (Increment in Muscle Mass) takes place, we observe decreased Fat percentage.

That means you are on Right Path; you are progressing and you should maintain the consistency and make further progression.

If we Consider Spiritual aspects as well:

In yoga and spirituality, it is said that, there are 5 important Vayus in the body. And out of them 'Udana Vayu' is important in consideration of weight. It's, main function is to carry anything upward and it's located in the region of Throat and Head. It maintains body's erect posture. And it counteracts Gravity. Imbalance of Udana Vayu affects, nervous health, respiratory problems, vocal cord and stubborn weight issues (could possibly be related to 'Thyroid Gland').

So finally, we have to consider only Fat percentage, in the fat also, we need to target the Visceral fat and maintain the neutral range of other two types of fats. And understand that, our body is going through a process of lifestyle change for good, so maintain this good lifestyle and make it a habit with patience.

And then expect the unexpected.

Importance of Fitness and Health

There are many things, which we may consider under this topic.

Being healthy should be part of your overall lifestyle. Living a healthy lifestyle can help prevent chronic diseases and long-term illnesses. Feeling good about yourself and taking care of your health are important for your self-esteem and self-image. Maintain a healthy lifestyle by doing what is right for your body.

Good health is central to human happiness and **well-being** that makes an **important** contribution to prosperity and wealth

Good health is an essential pre-requisite for the persistent and adequate functioning of an individual and a society.

Every part of your life relies on you having **good health**.

Health is a **positive concept emphasizing social and personal resources, as well as physical capacities**." This means that health is a resource to support an individual's function in wider society, rather than an end in itself. A healthful lifestyle provides the means to lead a full life with meaning and purpose.

Strengths and Weaknesses

Self-understanding:

Self-understanding refers to an individual's awareness and comprehension of their own values, beliefs, motivations, emotions, and behaviours. Understanding one's strengths and weaknesses is an important aspect of self-understanding as it provides insight into one's personal attributes and limitations.

Strengths refer to the positive traits, skills, and qualities that an individual possesses. These may include things like good communication skills, strong work ethic, creativity, leadership, and organization. Understanding one's strengths can help individuals leverage them to achieve their goals and feel more confident and capable in their personal and professional lives.

Weaknesses, on the other hand, are traits, habits, or areas where an individual may struggle or need improvement. Examples of weaknesses may include poor time management, procrastination, lack of confidence, and difficulty with public speaking. Understanding one's weaknesses can be challenging, as it often requires facing areas of personal challenge and growth. However, recognizing and addressing weaknesses can lead to personal growth and development.

It's important to keep in mind that strengths and weaknesses are not absolute and can change over time with experience and effort. Additionally, it's crucial to approach self-reflection with a growth mindset, recognizing that everyone has both strengths and weaknesses and that working on improving weaknesses can lead to personal growth and development. It's important to identify both strengths and weaknesses in fitness to set achievable goals, design an effective workout plan, and track progress over time. By focusing on improving weaknesses, individuals can become more well-rounded and improve their overall fitness level. Individuals can work to improve their overall fitness level, reduce their risk of injury, and perform better in physical activities. Additionally, focusing on areas of weakness can help prevent imbalances and promote overall health and wellness. Improving over weaknesses, individuals can become more well-rounded and physically prepared for a wider range of activities. Additionally, recognizing and addressing weaknesses can help prevent injury and promote overall health and wellness. It's important to keep in mind that fitness is a continuous process and it's always possible to improve upon strengths and overcome weaknesses.

Genetics and Fitness

Genetics and physical fitness are related in several ways. Here are some key aspects of this relationship:

1. **Inherited traits:** Physical fitness is influenced by many factors, including genetics. Inherited traits such as muscle fibre type, body composition, and metabolism can determine an individual's athletic potential and determine how efficiently their body processes energy, builds muscle, and burns fat.

2. **Genetic predispositions:** Some people may have a genetic predisposition to certain physical traits, such as increased muscle mass or improved endurance, which can make them more naturally inclined to excel in certain sports or activities. However, it is important to note that genetics is only one aspect of physical fitness and many other factors, such as training, nutrition, and lifestyle, also play a significant role.

3. **Genetic variations and performance:** Some genetic variations can have a direct impact on athletic performance. For example, a specific genetic mutation has been linked to improved endurance in long-distance runners. Similarly,

genetic variations in muscle fibres, metabolism, and other aspects of physiology can affect strength, power, and other aspects of athletic performance.

4. **Gene doping:** Some athletes attempt to enhance their performance by manipulating their genes. This is known as "gene doping" and is considered unethical and banned by many sports organizations.

5. **Personalized training and nutrition:** Understanding an individual's genetic background can also inform personalized training and nutrition programs, allowing athletes and fitness enthusiasts to optimize their workouts and diets to maximize their potential.

6. **Injury susceptibility:** Some genetic variations can increase the risk of certain types of injuries, such as ankle sprains or knee injuries. Understanding these genetic predispositions can help individuals take preventative measures to reduce their risk of injury.

7. **Recovery:** Genetics can also play a role in how quickly an individual recover from injury or intense physical activity. Some people may have genes that allow them to recover more quickly, while others may take longer.

8. **Physical activity tolerance:** Genetics can also influence how an individual tolerates physical activity. Some people may have a naturally higher tolerance for exercise and be able to handle intense physical activity without experiencing negative effects, while others may struggle with even moderate activity levels.

9. **Nutrient metabolism:** Nutrient metabolism is another area where genetics can play a role. Some people may have a genetic predisposition to process certain nutrients, such as carbohydrates or fat, more efficiently than others, which can affect their physical fitness and athletic performance.

10. **Environmental factors:** It is important to note that genetics is just one piece of the puzzle when it comes to physical fitness. Environmental factors, such as nutrition, physical activity, and lifestyle, can greatly impact an individual's physical fitness and athletic performance. For example, a person with a genetic predisposition to increased muscle mass may not see the benefits of that predisposition if they do not engage in regular strength training and adequate protein intake.

11. **Age-related decline:** Genetics can also play a role in how an individual's physical fitness and athletic performance changes with age. Some

people may experience a slower decline in physical fitness and athletic performance as they age, while others may experience a more rapid decline.

12. **Genetic disorders:** Certain genetic disorders, such as muscular dystrophy or Marfan syndrome, can greatly impact an individual's physical fitness and athletic performance. Understanding these disorders and their effects on the body can help individuals make informed decisions about their physical activity and exercise routines.

13. **Performance-enhancing drugs:** Performance-enhancing drugs, such as anabolic steroids, can also have a significant impact on physical fitness and athletic performance. However, it is important to note that these drugs can have serious health consequences and are often banned by sports organizations.

14. **Motivation and drive:** While genetics can play a role in physical fitness, motivation and drive are also important factors. Some individuals may be naturally more motivated to engage in physical activity and exercise, while others may need to work harder to develop this motivation.

15. **Mind-body connection:** The mind-body connection is another important aspect of the relationship between genetics and physical

fitness. Mental and emotional factors, such as stress and anxiety, can greatly impact an individual's physical fitness and athletic performance. By understanding the mind-body connection and the role that mental and emotional factors play in physical fitness, individuals can make informed decisions about their exercise and physical activity routines.

Genetics can play a role in determining physical fitness, but it is only one aspect of many that contribute to an individual's overall athletic potential. However, it is important to remember that genetics is not destiny, and that proper training, nutrition, and lifestyle can greatly impact physical fitness and athletic performance. Genetics and physical fitness are complexly interwoven and understanding the relationship between these two factors can help individuals make informed decisions about their physical fitness and athletic performance. While genetics can play a role, it is just one aspect of many that contribute to an individual's overall athletic potential and success.

Good Habits – Bad Habits

Good Habits:

1. **Regular Exercise:** Physical activity is important for maintaining a healthy body and mind. Engaging in regular exercise helps reduce the risk of chronic illnesses such as heart disease, obesity, and diabetes.

2. **Healthy Eating:** Eating a well-balanced and nutritious diet is essential for good health. A healthy diet should include plenty of fruits, vegetables, whole grains, lean proteins, and healthy fats.

3. **Sufficient Sleep:** Getting enough sleep is crucial for physical and mental health. Lack of sleep can lead to fatigue, mood swings, and decreased cognitive function.

4. **Time Management:** Managing time effectively is essential for achieving goals and reducing stress. Prioritizing tasks and setting achievable deadlines can help improve productivity.

5. **Positive Thinking:** Positive thinking is a key component of a healthy mindset. It can help reduce stress, boost self-esteem, and improve overall well-being.

Bad Habits:

1. **Sedentary Lifestyle:** A sedentary lifestyle, characterized by a lack of physical activity, can lead to a host of health problems including obesity, heart disease, and diabetes.

2. **Unhealthy Eating:** Consuming a diet that is high in processed foods, sugars, and unhealthy fats can lead to weight gain, high blood pressure, and other chronic illnesses.

3. **Inadequate Sleep:** Lack of sleep or poor sleep quality can lead to a range of health problems, including fatigue, mood swings, and decreased cognitive function.

4. **Procrastination:** Procrastination can lead to missed deadlines, increased stress, and decreased productivity. It can also make it difficult to achieve goals.

5. **Negative Thinking:** Negative thinking can lead to a range of mental health problems, including anxiety and depression. It can also affect physical health by increasing stress and reducing overall well-being.

How Bad habits or addictions can affect next generation, in terms of genetic information and DNA:

Bad habits or addictions can have both direct and indirect effects on the next generation.

Direct effects can occur if a parent engages in a behaviour that directly impacts their DNA, which can then be passed on to their offspring. For example, exposure to certain toxins, such as tobacco smoke, can cause changes in DNA that can be inherited by future generations. These changes can increase the risk of genetic mutations and diseases in offspring.

Indirect effects can occur through epigenetic mechanisms. Epigenetic changes are changes to the DNA that do not alter the genetic code itself but affect the expression of genes. Exposure to environmental factors, such as stress or substance abuse, can cause epigenetic changes that can be passed on to future generations. These changes can alter the expression of genes that play a role in brain development, behaviour, and addiction, increasing the risk of addiction and other behavioural problems in offspring.

Children of parents with addictions or bad habits may be more likely to adopt these behaviours themselves due to genetic predispositions, environmental factors, or learned behaviours. For example, children of parents who smoke are more likely to smoke themselves.

Genetics and DNA are only one factor in the development of addiction and bad habits. Environmental factors, such as social and cultural influences, also play a significant role. It is possible to break the cycle of addiction and bad habits through early intervention, education, and treatment.

Here are some examples of how bad habits or addictions can affect the next generation:

1. **Alcoholism:** Children of alcoholic parents are at higher risk of developing alcoholism themselves. This increased risk is partly due to genetic factors, as there are specific genes that have been linked to alcoholism. However, environmental factors, such as parental modelling of drinking behaviours and exposure to stress and trauma, also play a significant role.

2. **Smoking:** Children of parents who smoke are more likely to start smoking themselves. This increased risk is due to both genetic and environmental factors. For example, genetic factors can influence nicotine metabolism and addiction, while environmental factors such as parental modelling and exposure to second-hand smoke can also play a role.

3. **Drug addiction:** Children of parents with a history of drug addiction are at higher risk of developing addiction themselves. This increased risk is due to both genetic and environmental factors, as drug addiction has been shown to have a strong genetic component, but environmental factors such as parental

modelling and exposure to stress and trauma also play a significant role.

4. **Unhealthy eating habits:** Children of parents who have poor eating habits or who consume a diet high in processed foods and unhealthy fats may be more likely to develop obesity, diabetes, and other health problems. This increased risk is due to both genetic and environmental factors, as there are specific genes that have been linked to obesity and metabolic disorders, but environmental factors such as parental modelling and access to healthy foods also play a role.

5. **Workaholism:** Children of workaholic parents may be more likely to develop workaholic tendencies themselves, leading to a range of negative effects on their health and well-being. This increased risk is due to environmental factors such as parental modelling of workaholic behaviours and exposure to stress and pressure to succeed.

6. **Gambling addiction:** Children of parents with gambling addictions are at higher risk of developing gambling problems themselves. This increased risk is due to both genetic and environmental factors, as there are specific genes that have been linked to gambling addiction, but environmental factors such as

parental modelling and exposure to gambling behaviours also play a role.

7. **Technology addiction:** Children of parents who excessively use technology, such as smartphones or social media, may be more likely to develop problematic technology use themselves. This increased risk is due to environmental factors, such as parental modelling of technology use and exposure to screens from an early age.

8. **Anger management problems:** Children of parents with anger management problems may be more likely to develop similar problems themselves. This increased risk is due to both genetic and environmental factors, as there are specific genes that have been linked to aggression and anger, but environmental factors such as parental modelling of aggressive behaviours and exposure to stressful or violent environments also play a role.

9. **Exercise addiction:** Children of parents with exercise addictions may be more likely to develop similar problems themselves. This increased risk is due to both genetic and environmental factors, as there are specific genes that have been linked to exercise addiction, but environmental factors such as parental modelling of excessive exercise

behaviours and pressure to excel in sports or fitness may also play a role.

10. **Chronic stress:** Children of parents who experience chronic stress may be more likely to develop similar problems themselves. This increased risk is due to environmental factors, such as exposure to stressful environments and parental modelling of stress management strategies. Chronic stress has been linked to a range of health problems, including depression, anxiety, and cardiovascular disease.

Age and Fitness

Age is a major factor that affects physical fitness. As people grow older, various physiological changes occur that can affect their physical fitness.

1. **Decreased muscle mass and strength:** With age, there is a gradual loss of muscle mass and strength, known as sarcopenia. This results in a decrease in physical performance, making it more difficult to perform physical activities.
2. **Decreased flexibility:** As people age, their joints and muscles become less flexible, making it harder to perform movements that require a full range of motion, such as bending and reaching. This can also increase the risk of injury.
3. **Decreased cardiovascular fitness:** The heart and blood vessels also undergo changes with age, leading to a decrease in cardiovascular fitness. This can result in decreased endurance and increased fatigue during physical activity.
4. **Decreased balance and coordination:** As people age, their balance and coordination can decline, increasing the risk of falls and other accidents.

However, these changes do not have to occur at the same rate for everyone. Physical fitness can be maintained and improved at any age through regular physical activity, such as resistance training and cardiovascular exercise. Staying physically active can help to slow down the aging process, reduce the risk of chronic diseases, and improve overall quality of life.

It's important to note that while age can affect physical fitness, other factors such as genetics, lifestyle, and past physical activity also play a role. So, while physical fitness may decline with age, it is possible to maintain and even improve physical fitness with proper exercise and a healthy lifestyle.

There are also various other factors that can influence physical fitness levels. Some of these factors include:

1. **Nutrition:** A balanced diet that provides the necessary nutrients and energy to support physical activity is essential for maintaining physical fitness.
2. **Sleep:** Adequate sleep is important for recovery and repair of the body after physical activity, and can help improve physical performance.
3. **Stress:** Chronic stress can have a negative impact on physical fitness by affecting the body's ability to recover from physical activity and increasing the risk of injury.

4. **Genetics:** Certain genetic factors can influence physical fitness levels, such as muscle mass, endurance, and the body's ability to use oxygen efficiently.
5. **Smoking:** Smoking has a negative impact on physical fitness by affecting lung function, cardiovascular health, and muscle strength.
6. **Chronic diseases:** Chronic diseases such as diabetes, heart disease, and arthritis can affect physical fitness levels and the ability to participate in physical activity.

It is important to take a holistic approach to maintaining physical fitness by considering all of these factors, and not just age. Regular physical activity, a balanced diet, adequate sleep, stress management, and avoiding behaviours such as smoking can all help to maintain and improve physical fitness throughout life. Seek an Expert's advice before starting any new physical activity, especially if you have any existing health conditions. This is particularly important for older adults, who may have more health concerns and may require modifications to their physical activity routine.

Incorporating a variety of physical activities into your routine can help to maintain and improve physical fitness. This can include aerobic exercise, such as jogging or cycling, to improve cardiovascular fitness, resistance training, such as weightlifting, to build muscle strength and mass, and flexibility exercises, such as yoga or stretching, to improve range of motion and reduce the risk of injury. The relationship between age and physical fitness is complex and can be influenced by a variety of factors. However, with regular physical activity, a balanced diet, adequate sleep, and stress management, it is possible to maintain and even improve physical fitness throughout life, regardless of age.

Oxidative Stress

Oxidative stress is a condition that occurs when there is an imbalance between the production of reactive oxygen species (ROS) and the ability of cells to detoxify them or repair the resulting damage. ROS are chemically reactive molecules that are produced as by-products of normal cellular metabolism and also in response to various environmental stressors, such as ultraviolet radiation, pollution, and cigarette smoke.

Under normal conditions, cells have antioxidant defence mechanisms to neutralize ROS and prevent damage to cellular components such as DNA, proteins, and lipids. However, when there is an excess of ROS or a deficiency in antioxidant defences, oxidative stress can occur, leading to cellular damage and dysfunction.

Oxidative stress has been implicated in a wide range of diseases, including cancer, cardiovascular disease, neurodegenerative disorders such as Alzheimer's and Parkinson's disease, and inflammatory conditions such as rheumatoid arthritis. In these diseases, oxidative stress can lead to DNA damage, protein cross-linking, and lipid peroxidation, which can ultimately lead to cell death or dysfunction.

Oxidative stress occurs when there is an imbalance between the production of reactive oxygen species

(ROS) and the ability of cells to detoxify them or repair the resulting damage. ROS are chemically reactive molecules that are produced as by-products of normal cellular metabolism and also in response to various environmental stressors, such as ultraviolet radiation, pollution, and cigarette smoke.

ROS can be harmful to cells because they can react with and damage cellular components such as DNA, proteins, and lipids. This can lead to mutations in DNA, cross-linking of proteins, and lipid peroxidation, which can ultimately lead to cell death or dysfunction.

Under normal conditions, cells have antioxidant defence mechanisms to neutralize ROS and prevent damage to cellular components. Antioxidants are molecules that can donate an electron to ROS, thereby neutralizing them and preventing them from causing damage. Some examples of antioxidants include vitamin C, vitamin E, and glutathione.

However, when there is an excess of ROS or a deficiency in antioxidant defences, oxidative stress can occur. This can happen in several ways. For example, exposure to environmental toxins such as cigarette smoke can overwhelm the body's antioxidant defences, leading to oxidative stress. Similarly, chronic inflammation can also produce an excess of ROS, leading to oxidative stress.

Lifestyle factors such as a poor diet, lack of exercise, and exposure to toxins can also contribute to oxidative stress. A diet that is high in processed foods and low in fruits and vegetables can lead to a deficiency in antioxidants, which can contribute to oxidative stress. Similarly, a sedentary lifestyle can reduce the body's antioxidant defences, while exposure to environmental toxins such as air pollution can increase the production of ROS.

Lifestyle and Fitness

Lifestyle and fitness are closely related and interconnected concepts. A person's lifestyle greatly affects their overall health and fitness. A healthy lifestyle includes regular physical activity, a balanced diet, stress management, and adequate sleep, among other things. All of these factors play a crucial role in maintaining a person's overall physical and mental well-being.

On the other hand, a sedentary lifestyle, characterized by lack of physical activity and poor dietary choices, can lead to health problems such as obesity, heart disease, and type 2 diabetes. Engaging in regular physical activity and adopting a healthy diet can help mitigate the negative effects of a sedentary lifestyle and improve overall health and fitness.

Lifestyle and fitness are intertwined, and one greatly affects the other. Adopting a healthy lifestyle can lead to improved fitness levels, while being fit can help support and maintain a healthy lifestyle.

Fitness goals can play a significant role in shaping a person's lifestyle. For example, a person who has a goal of running a marathon may need to make changes to their lifestyle, such as increasing their physical activity, eating a balanced diet, and getting enough sleep, to achieve their goal.

Fitness can also impact mental health and well-being. Regular physical activity has been shown to boost mood, reduce stress, and improve cognitive function. These benefits can then have a positive impact on other aspects of a person's life, such as work and relationships.

The relationship between lifestyle and fitness is a two-way street. A person's lifestyle affects their fitness level, and their fitness goals and level of physical activity can also shape their lifestyle choices. By prioritizing a healthy lifestyle and regular physical activity, a person can improve their overall health and well-being, both physically and mentally.

Another aspect to consider is that lifestyle habits can have both short-term and long-term effects on fitness. For example, regularly skipping meals or engaging in binge eating can lead to immediate changes in energy levels and weight, but it can also lead to long-term health problems, such as heart disease and type 2 diabetes. On the other hand, incorporating healthy habits into your daily routine, such as eating a balanced diet and engaging in physical activity, can lead to immediate benefits, such as improved mood and increased energy levels, as well as long-term benefits, such as a lower risk of chronic diseases.

A healthy lifestyle and fitness aren't just about avoiding negative health outcomes. They also contribute to overall well-being and quality of life. Engaging in physical activity and adopting healthy habits can lead to improved self-esteem, better sleep, and a more positive outlook on life.

The relationship between lifestyle and fitness is complex and multifaceted. By making choices that support a healthy lifestyle, a person can improve their fitness level and overall well-being, both in the short-term and the long-term.

Immunity and Exercise

Exercise and immunity are closely related, as physical activity can impact the body's immune system in several ways. Here are some of the ways exercise affects immunity:

1. **Boosts immune function:** Regular exercise has been shown to improve the function of the immune system, particularly by increasing the production of white blood cells, which help fight off infections and diseases.

2. **Reduces inflammation:** Exercise can reduce inflammation in the body, which is a key factor in many diseases and health conditions. Chronic inflammation can weaken the immune system, but physical activity can help keep it under control.

3. **Stress reduction:** Exercise can also help reduce stress, which can weaken the immune system. Chronic stress can lead to a decrease in the number and activity of white blood cells, making the body more susceptible to illness and infection.

4. **Improves sleep:** Exercise has been shown to improve sleep quality, which is important for immune function. Adequate sleep is essential

for the body to repair and regenerate, including the immune system.

5. **Promotes lymphatic circulation:** Exercise can help stimulate lymphatic circulation, which is crucial for the immune system. The lymphatic system is responsible for filtering out waste and debris, and for transporting immune cells throughout the body.

6. **Increases antioxidant levels:** Exercise can increase the levels of antioxidants in the body, which protect against oxidative stress and help keep the immune system functioning properly.

7. **Increases metabolism:** Regular exercise can also increase metabolism, which can help improve overall health and boost the immune system.

8. **Supports gut health:** The gut is home to a large part of the body's immune system, and exercise has been shown to support gut health by promoting the growth of beneficial bacteria and reducing inflammation.

9. **Supports mental health:** Exercise has been shown to have a positive impact on mental health, which in turn can help boost immunity. Mental stress and anxiety can weaken the immune system, and physical activity can help reduce these negative effects.

10. **May improve chronic illness outcomes:** Certain chronic illnesses, such as diabetes and heart disease, can weaken the immune system. Regular exercise has been shown to improve outcomes for these conditions, which can in turn help support immune function.
11. **Supports healthy aging:** As we age, the immune system can become less effective, making us more susceptible to illness and infection. Regular exercise has been shown to support healthy aging and help maintain a strong and functional immune system.
12. **Aids in weight management:** Maintaining a healthy weight is important for immune function, and regular exercise can help with weight management. Obesity has been linked to a weakened immune system and increased risk of certain illnesses, so staying active can help reduce these risks.

Exercise plays a crucial role in supporting immune function and overall health. Regular physical activity can boost immunity, reduce inflammation, improve sleep and mental health, support healthy aging, aid in weight management, and more. It's important to listen to your body and engage in regular physical activity in moderation for the best results.

However, it's important to note that excessive or intense exercise can have the opposite effect, and weaken the immune system by causing oxidative stress and inflammation. This is why moderation is key when it comes to exercise and immunity. Regular moderate exercise is generally beneficial for the immune system, while excessive or intense exercise can have negative effects.

Exercise is an important component of a healthy lifestyle and can have a positive impact on the immune system. Regular physical activity can boost immune function, reduce inflammation, improve sleep, and support overall health, among other benefits. However, it's important to listen to your body and not overdo it, as excessive or intense exercise can have negative effects on the immune system.

Beauty in Simplicity

"Beauty in Simplicity" in fitness refers to the idea that achieving optimal fitness and health can be attained through simple and sustainable actions, rather than complex and restrictive methods.

It emphasizes the importance of focusing on basic and fundamental principles of fitness, such as regular exercise, a balanced and nutritious diet, adequate sleep, and stress management, instead of constantly seeking out the latest fad or trend.

By keeping things simple and manageable, individuals can more easily integrate healthy habits into their daily lives and maintain them in the long term, leading to improved physical and mental well-being. Choosing exercises that are simple and effective, rather than complicated or trendy. Instead of constantly seeking out new and complex exercises or workout routines, focusing on fundamental movements such as squats, lunges, push-ups, and pull-ups can be highly effective for building strength, improving mobility, and enhancing overall fitness. Furthermore, emphasizing compound exercises that work multiple muscle groups simultaneously can be more efficient and effective than isolated exercises that target only one muscle group. By selecting simple yet effective exercises that can be easily integrated into a regular fitness routine, individuals can achieve their fitness goals more efficiently, while also reducing the risk of injury and maintaining motivation over time.

Minimally processed foods that are simple and nutritious, rather than constantly seeking out complicated or restrictive diet plans. By emphasizing whole foods such as fruits, vegetables, lean proteins, whole grains, and healthy fats, individuals can obtain a balanced and varied nutrient intake, which can improve overall health and reduce the risk of chronic diseases. Simplifying one's diet can also make it easier to maintain a healthy and sustainable eating pattern in the long term, as it reduces the need for calorie counting or strict meal planning. Rather than relying on complex or trendy diets, focusing on a varied and balanced diet that incorporates simple, whole foods can provide numerous health benefits, while also being easier to sustain over time.

Give sufficient required Time and Keep Patience

Time and patience are essential in any fitness journey for several reasons:

1. **Sustainable progress:** Fitness is a long-term journey, and it takes time to see meaningful progress. With patience, you can avoid the temptation to rush and give up early, which can lead to unsustainable results.
2. **Avoid injuries:** Rushing into fitness can lead to injuries. Taking time to build a solid foundation of strength and endurance while gradually increasing intensity can help you avoid injuries.
3. **Mental health:** Patience in fitness helps you develop mental strength and resilience. With time, you learn to appreciate the process and enjoy the journey, which can improve your mental health.
4. **Lifestyle change:** Building a healthy lifestyle takes time, and it requires patience to change your habits gradually.
5. **Consistency:** Consistency is key in fitness. By committing to a fitness routine over time and allowing for patience, you can create a habit and make it a part of your lifestyle. This consistency

can help you achieve long-term goals and maintain good health.

6. **Plateaus:** It's common to hit a plateau in fitness, where progress seems to stall. Patience and persistence are crucial to push through this stage, as it can take time for the body to adapt and see results again.

7. **Risk of burnout:** Trying to achieve results too quickly can lead to burnout and loss of motivation. Patience allows you to pace yourself and avoid feeling overwhelmed, making it more likely that you will continue to exercise and make progress.

Time and patience are essential in a fitness journey for numerous reasons, including sustainable progress, avoiding injuries, mental health, lifestyle change, consistency, pushing through plateaus, and avoiding burnout. Remember that fitness is a journey, not a destination, and by allowing time and being patient, you can achieve your goals and maintain good health for the long term.

Patience in fitness refers to the willingness to stick to a long-term exercise and nutrition plan without getting discouraged by slow progress or setbacks. It means understanding that sustainable results take time and consistency, and that there are no shortcuts or quick fixes. Practicing patience in fitness can help individuals avoid injury, prevent burnout, and maintain motivation to reach their goals. It involves setting realistic expectations, tracking progress, celebrating small victories, and staying committed to a healthy lifestyle even when progress may seem slow.

Patience in fitness can also mean being mindful of your body's limitations and respecting them. Overexerting yourself, pushing too hard too fast, or expecting rapid results can lead to injury or burnout, which can set you back even further. Practicing patience involves allowing yourself time to rest and recover, as well as being patient with the ups and downs that come with any fitness journey. It requires a long-term perspective, recognizing that health and fitness are not just short-term goals, but a continuous journey. It means making small, sustainable lifestyle changes that can be maintained over time, rather than going on extreme diets or exercise regimens that are difficult to sustain. Ultimately, patience in fitness means having a positive and realistic mindset that focuses on progress rather than perfection, and recognizes that sustainable change takes time and effort.

Consistency, Discipline and Progression

Consistency in fitness refers to regularly engaging in physical activity and maintaining a healthy lifestyle over time. This can include activities such as exercising, eating a balanced diet, and getting enough sleep.

Consistency is important in fitness because it allows for gradual progress and adaptation, leading to long-term improvements in physical health and well-being. By making physical activity and healthy habits a regular part of one's routine, it becomes easier to maintain progress and avoid setbacks.

Discipline in fitness involves adhering to a plan or routine in order to achieve specific fitness goals. This can include following a structured workout program, tracking progress, and adjusting as necessary.

Discipline is important because it provides structure and motivation for achieving fitness goals. It requires commitment and dedication to a plan, even when it may be difficult or uncomfortable. By following a structured routine and tracking progress, individuals can monitor their results and adjust their approach to ensure continued progress.

Progression in fitness means gradually increasing the intensity, duration, or frequency of physical activity in order to continue making progress and achieving fitness goals. This can involve increasing weights or reps, adding new exercises, or challenging oneself in new ways to avoid plateaus and continue improving.

Progression is important because it challenges the body to adapt and improve over time. As the body becomes accustomed to a certain level of physical activity, it requires increased stimulus in order to continue making progress. By gradually increasing the intensity, duration, or frequency of physical activity, individuals can continue to challenge their body and achieve higher levels of fitness. However, it is important to progress gradually and safely to avoid injury and overtraining.

Expect from a consistent, disciplined and progressive fitness routine:

A consistent, disciplined, and progressive fitness routine can lead to improved physical health, increased strength and endurance, better body composition, increased energy levels, improved mood and mental health, better sleep quality, reduced risk of chronic diseases, and overall better quality of life.

Here's more in-depth information on what to expect from a consistent, disciplined, and progressive fitness routine:

1. **Improved Physical Health:** Regular exercise can lead to improved cardiovascular health, increased lung capacity, better blood pressure, improved digestion, and reduced risk of various health conditions like diabetes, heart disease, and certain types of cancer.

2. **Increased Strength and Endurance:** A consistent fitness routine that includes strength training can lead to increased muscle strength, endurance, and bone density. This can help prevent injuries and improve overall physical function.

3. **Better Body Composition:** Exercise can help reduce body fat, increase muscle mass, and improve overall body composition. This can lead to a more toned, fit, and healthy appearance.

4. **Increased Energy Levels:** Regular physical activity can improve energy levels, reduce fatigue, and boost overall productivity and alertness.

5. **Improved Mood and Mental Health:** Exercise can boost the production of endorphins, the body's natural feel-good chemicals, which can help reduce stress, anxiety, and depression.

6. **Better Sleep Quality:** Regular exercise can improve sleep quality, helping individuals fall asleep faster and stay asleep longer.

7. **Reduced Risk of Chronic Diseases:** A consistent fitness routine can reduce the risk of various chronic diseases like diabetes, heart disease, and some cancers. Exercise can also help manage existing health conditions like arthritis and high blood pressure.

A consistent, disciplined, and progressive fitness routine can have numerous physical, mental, and emotional health benefits that can help individuals achieve a better quality of life.

Realistic Fitness Goal

Realistic fitness goals are specific, achievable targets that consider your starting point, lifestyle, and abilities. They are grounded in reality, rather than wishful thinking, and allow you to make progress toward a healthier, more active lifestyle at a pace that suits you. Realistic fitness goals can help you stay motivated, avoid frustration and burnout, and achieve sustainable, long-term results. Examples of realistic fitness goals might include aiming to exercise for 30 minutes a day, 3-4 times a week, or to gradually increase your running distance or weightlifting reps over a period of several weeks.

Setting realistic fitness goals is an important step towards achieving a healthier, more active lifestyle. Realistic fitness goals are targets that are achievable and specific, considering your starting point, lifestyle, and abilities. These goals are grounded in reality, rather than wishful thinking, and allow you to make progress at a pace that suits you.

To set realistic fitness goals, you first need to determine your starting point. This might involve assessing your current level of fitness, identifying any health issues that could affect your ability to exercise, and understanding the demands of your lifestyle. From there, you can set specific, measurable goals that consider your personal circumstances and abilities.

Realistic fitness goals should also be achievable. While it's important to challenge yourself, setting goals that are too ambitious can lead to frustration and burnout. To avoid this, start by setting small, achievable goals that you can build on over time. For example, if you're new to exercise, you might set a goal to walk for 20 minutes a day, three days a week. Once you've achieved this, you can gradually increase the duration or frequency of your walks.

It's also important to be flexible with your fitness goals. Life can be unpredictable, and there may be times when you're unable to exercise as much as you'd like. If you've set a realistic fitness goal, you'll be better able to adapt to changes in your circumstances and stay on track.

Finally, realistic fitness goals should be relevant to your overall health and well-being. Rather than setting goals based on external factors such as appearance or societal pressure, focus on goals that will improve your physical and mental health. This might include goals related to strength, endurance, flexibility, or stress reduction.

Setting realistic fitness goals is an important step towards achieving a healthier, more active lifestyle. By setting specific, achievable, and relevant goals, you can stay motivated, avoid frustration and burnout, and achieve sustainable, long-term results.

Unrealistic Fitness Goals

Unrealistic fitness goals refer to health and fitness objectives that are extremely difficult or nearly impossible to achieve within a reasonable timeframe or without sacrificing overall health and well-being. Unrealistic fitness goals often result in frustration, disappointment, and a lack of motivation to continue pursuing fitness.

Examples of unrealistic fitness goals may include losing an unrealistic amount of weight within a short period of time, achieving an impossibly low body fat percentage, or completing a marathon without sufficient training. These types of goals can be harmful to physical and mental health and can result in injury, burnout, and a negative body image.

It is important to set achievable and sustainable fitness goals that are specific, measurable, realistic, and time-bound. This involves setting realistic expectations, creating a plan, tracking progress, and celebrating small successes along the way. By setting achievable fitness goals, individuals can maintain motivation and see sustainable progress toward their overall health and wellness goals.

Setting unrealistic fitness goals can have a detrimental effect on an individual's physical and mental health.

When people set goals that are too ambitious or unreasonable, they may end up feeling disappointed or frustrated when they don't achieve them. This can lead to a negative cycle of self-doubt, guilt, and stress that may impact their overall health and well-being.

Furthermore, unrealistic fitness goals can result in injury, especially when they involve extreme or rapid changes to an individual's fitness routine or diet. Attempting to lose a large amount of weight in a short period of time, for example, may require an unhealthy and unsustainable diet or exercise regimen that can cause physical harm.

To avoid unrealistic fitness goals, it is essential to focus on setting achievable and sustainable goals that align with an individual's lifestyle, physical abilities, and long-term aspirations. By setting SMART goals (specific, measurable, achievable, relevant, and time-bound), individuals can create a clear roadmap to success that is both challenging and realistic.

For example, a realistic fitness goal might be to lose 1-2 pounds per week, which is a safe and sustainable rate of weight loss. Alternatively, a goal might be to complete a 5k run within six months, which is a reasonable and achievable timeframe for most beginners. By setting achievable and realistic goals, individuals can stay motivated, track progress, and ultimately achieve their desired outcomes while maintaining good health and well-being.

Types of Recoveries

There are 3 types of recoveries:

1. **Immediate recovery:** This type of recovery occurs within minutes after the end of the workout. During this time, the body's metabolic rate and energy expenditure decrease rapidly as the heart rate and breathing rate begin to slow down. It is important to allow your body to cool down gradually and perform stretching exercises to prevent injury and reduce muscle soreness.

2. **Short-term recovery:** This type of recovery occurs in the hours and days following a workout. During this time, the body repairs damaged muscle fibers, replenishes glycogen stores, and removes waste products such as lactic acid. Adequate nutrition, including protein and carbohydrates, and hydration are important to support muscle recovery during this phase. Sleep is also important for muscle recovery as growth hormone, which is responsible for muscle repair and growth, is released during deep sleep.

3. **Long-term recovery:** This type of recovery occurs over the course of several weeks to

several months. It is important to allow the body to fully recover and adapt to the demands of the training program during this phase to prevent overtraining and injury. During this time, the body may also benefit from a period of active rest, which involves reducing the intensity or volume of workouts to allow the body to recover while still maintaining fitness. Proper nutrition, hydration, and sleep are critical during this phase to support the body's recovery and adaptation.

Apart from these types there are another form of recovery:

> A) **Active Recovery:** Active recovery refers to the use of low-intensity exercise or movement as a means of aiding the recovery process following more intense or strenuous physical activity. It involves engaging in activities that help to stimulate circulation, promote relaxation, reduce muscle soreness, and prevent stiffness. Active recovery can also help to promote mental and emotional well-being by reducing stress and tension in the body.

Active recovery is often recommended for athletes, fitness enthusiasts, and individuals who engage in high-intensity exercise or physical activity on a regular basis. The purpose of active recovery is to help the body recover from the stress and strain of exercise, while also preventing injury and promoting overall health and well-being.

Some examples of activities that may be used for active recovery include:

1. **Light jogging or walking:** This can help to stimulate circulation and promote the flow of oxygen and nutrients to the muscles.
2. **Yoga or stretching:** This can help to reduce muscle soreness, improve flexibility, and promote relaxation.
3. **Swimming:** This can help to reduce the impact on joints and muscles, while also promoting cardiovascular health.
4. **Cycling:** This can help to improve blood flow, reduce muscle soreness, and provide a low-impact workout.
5. **Foam rolling:** This involves using a foam roller to apply pressure to specific areas of the body, which can help to reduce muscle tension and soreness.

It is important to note that active recovery should be performed at a low intensity, as the goal is to aid in the recovery process, rather than to engage in more intense exercise. It is also important to listen to your body and adjust your active recovery routine as needed based on your level of fatigue or soreness.

Active recovery is a useful technique for promoting recovery and reducing muscle soreness following intense physical activity. By engaging in low-intensity exercise or movement, individuals can help to stimulate circulation, reduce muscle tension, and promote overall health and well-being

> B) **Passive Recovery:** Passive recovery refers to a type of recovery strategy that involves resting and allowing the body to recover naturally, without engaging in any structured exercise or activity. This approach to recovery is often used by athletes and fitness enthusiasts to help the body recover from intense training or competition.

Passive recovery can take many different forms, but it generally involves some combination of the following:

1. **Rest:** This is the most basic component of passive recovery, and it simply involves taking time off from training or physical activity. This

allows the body to rest and recuperate, which can help reduce muscle soreness and fatigue.

2. **Sleep:** Getting enough sleep is essential for recovery, as it is during sleep that the body repairs and rebuilds damaged tissues. It is recommended that adults get between 7-9 hours of sleep per night.

3. **Hydration:** Staying hydrated is important for recovery, as it helps flush out toxins and waste products that can build up in the body during intense exercise. Drinking plenty of water and other fluids can help speed up the recovery process.

4. **Nutrition:** Eating a healthy, balanced diet is essential for recovery, as it provides the body with the nutrients it needs to repair and rebuild tissues. Consuming foods high in protein, carbohydrates, and antioxidants can help speed up the recovery process.

5. **Stretching:** Gentle stretching can help alleviate muscle soreness and stiffness, and can help improve flexibility and range of motion. This can be particularly helpful after intense exercise or competition.

6. **Massage:** Massage can help improve blood flow and reduce muscle tension, which can help speed up the recovery process. This can be done

by a professional massage therapist or by using a foam roller or other self-massage tools.

Passive recovery can be particularly useful after intense exercise or competition, as it allows the body to recover naturally and can help reduce the risk of injury or burnout. However, it is important to note that passive recovery should not be used as a substitute for proper training and exercise, and that it is important to maintain a balance between activity and rest in order to achieve optimal health and fitness.

Importance of Stretches in recovery

Stretches play a crucial role in recovery, both after a workout and in general. Stretching involves deliberately elongating and lengthening your muscles to improve flexibility and mobility. The act of stretching not only helps to alleviate muscle tension and soreness, but it also improves blood flow, which can aid in the recovery process.

Here are some specific ways in which stretching is important for recovery:

1. **Improving Flexibility:** Stretching increases your range of motion, which can help to prevent injury and make daily movements easier. When your muscles are flexible, they are less likely to become strained or pulled, allowing you to perform at your best during workouts and activities.

2. **Decreasing Muscle Tension:** After an intense workout, your muscles can feel tight and tense. Stretching can help to alleviate this tension, promoting relaxation and improving your overall mood. When you feel less tense, you are less likely to experience stiffness and soreness, which can help you recover more quickly.

3. **Enhancing Blood Flow:** Stretching improves blood circulation, which is essential for delivering oxygen and nutrients to your muscles. Increased blood flow can help to reduce inflammation and promote the removal of waste products such as lactic acid, which can contribute to muscle soreness and fatigue.

4. **Preventing Injury:** By improving your flexibility and reducing muscle tension, stretching can help to prevent injury. Tight muscles are more susceptible to strains and pulls, while flexible muscles are better able to withstand stress and strain.

5. **Promoting Relaxation:** Stretching can help to promote relaxation and reduce stress, which can be beneficial for both physical and mental recovery. When you feel less stressed and more relaxed, you are better able to focus on your recovery and prepare for your next workout or activity.

Stretching is an essential component of recovery. Whether you are an athlete or simply looking to improve your overall health and wellness, incorporating stretching into your routine can help you feel better, recover more quickly, and perform at your best.

Lactic Acid and its effect on recovery

During intense exercise, your body needs to generate energy to sustain the high level of activity. This energy is mainly produced through a process called glycolysis, which breaks down glucose (carbohydrates) into pyruvate. Under normal conditions, pyruvate is then transported into the mitochondria, where it enters the aerobic energy production cycle.

However, during high-intensity exercise, the demand for energy production exceeds the supply of oxygen to the muscle cells. As a result, pyruvate is converted into lactic acid through a process called anaerobic glycolysis. This conversion is catalysed by an enzyme called lactate dehydrogenase.

The accumulation of lactic acid in muscles leads to an increase in acidity (a decrease in pH), which can cause fatigue and a burning sensation. This happens because the acidity inhibits enzymes that are essential for energy production, which in turn leads to a reduction in muscle contraction and ultimately to exhaustion.

The body has a variety of mechanisms to remove lactic acid from the muscles and blood. One way is to transport it out of the muscle cells into the bloodstream, where it can be transported to the liver and converted back into glucose through a process called gluconeogenesis. Another way is to oxidize it in the mitochondria of the heart and other organs that can use lactic acid as a fuel source.

If lactic acid stays in the blood and muscles for an extended period, it can lead to delayed onset muscle soreness (DOMS), which is the pain and stiffness felt in muscles several hours after exercise. This is because lactic acid can cause inflammation and damage to muscle fibres, which triggers an immune response and leads to the release of chemicals that cause pain and soreness.

Lactic acid formation is a natural by-product of high-intensity exercise, and it plays a crucial role in energy production. However, the accumulation of lactic acid can lead to fatigue, muscle soreness, and decreased performance. The body has mechanisms to remove lactic acid from the muscles and blood, but if it stays in the body for an extended period, it can cause damage and delay recovery.

In addition to the mechanisms mentioned above, there are several other factors that can affect lactic acid formation and removal during exercise, which can ultimately impact recovery.

One such factor is the intensity and duration of the exercise. Higher intensity exercise leads to greater lactic acid accumulation, while longer duration exercise leads to more time for the body to remove lactic acid. Additionally, the type of exercise can also impact lactic acid formation, as certain types of exercise, such as high-intensity interval training, are known to produce higher levels of lactic acid than others.

Other factors that can affect lactic acid formation and removal include the individual's fitness level, age, diet, and hydration status. For example, individuals with higher fitness levels may be able to produce and remove lactic acid more efficiently than those with lower fitness levels. Similarly, a diet that is high in carbohydrates can provide the necessary fuel for energy production and help prevent lactic acid accumulation.

To optimize recovery and minimize muscle soreness, it is important to engage in proper cool-down and stretching after exercise, stay hydrated, and maintain a balanced diet that supports energy production and recovery. Additionally, massage, foam rolling, and other recovery techniques can help promote blood flow and reduce inflammation, which can aid in the removal of lactic acid and promote faster recovery.

Matured Perspective towards Health and Fitness

Maintaining a mature perspective towards health and fitness involves recognizing the importance of taking care of your body and mind throughout your life, and adopting healthy habits that are sustainable over the long term. Here are some key aspects of a mature perspective towards health and fitness:

1. **Consistency:** A mature perspective towards health and fitness recognizes that it is important to establish consistent habits that can be maintained over time. This means creating a daily or weekly routine that includes healthy habits such as regular exercise, a balanced diet, sufficient sleep, and stress management practices.

2. **Moderation:** Moderation is key when it comes to health and fitness. A mature perspective recognizes that extreme or unsustainable diets or exercise routines can be harmful to the body and can lead to burnout. Instead, a balanced approach that includes a variety of physical activities and a diverse diet is more likely to lead to sustainable long-term health and fitness.

3. **Mind-body connection:** A mature perspective towards health and fitness recognizes the connection between physical health and mental health. Engaging in regular physical activity can have a positive impact on mental health, reducing stress and anxiety, while practicing mindfulness and other mental health techniques can also support physical health.
4. **Prevention:** A mature perspective towards health and fitness recognizes the importance of preventive measures to maintain good health over time. This includes things like getting regular check-ups and screenings, practicing safe sex, wearing sunscreen, and avoiding harmful substances like tobacco and excessive alcohol.
5. **Individuality:** A mature perspective towards health and fitness recognizes that everyone's needs are different. What works for one person may not work for another. Therefore, it is important to listen to your body and find what works for you in terms of physical activity, diet, and other health practices.
6. **Lifelong learning:** A mature perspective towards health and fitness recognizes that there is always more to learn. New research is constantly emerging on health and fitness, and

it is important to stay up to date and incorporate new knowledge into your health practices.

7. **Flexibility:** Finally, a mature perspective towards health and fitness recognizes that life is unpredictable and that it is important to be flexible in your approach. This means being willing to adjust your routines and habits as needed to accommodate changes in your lifestyle, health status, and other factors that may affect your health and fitness.

8. **Setting realistic goals:** A mature perspective towards health and fitness involves setting realistic and achievable goals. Rather than setting overly ambitious goals that are difficult to reach, it is important to set small, achievable goals that can be built upon over time. This helps to build confidence and motivation, and creates a positive feedback loop that encourages continued progress.

9. **Seeking professional advice:** A mature perspective towards health and fitness involves recognizing when it is important to seek professional advice. This may include consulting with a doctor, nutritionist, or personal trainer to develop a personalized plan for your health and fitness. It is also important to recognize the value of professional support

for issues related to mental health, stress, and other related concerns.

10. **Emphasizing health over appearance:** A mature perspective towards health and fitness involves recognizing that the ultimate goal is to maintain good health, rather than achieving a certain appearance. This means focusing on developing healthy habits that support overall health and wellbeing, rather than engaging in unhealthy behaviours in pursuit of a specific body type or aesthetic.

11. **Being patient:** A mature perspective towards health and fitness involves recognizing that progress takes time, and that it is important to be patient with yourself throughout the process. Rather than expecting immediate results, it is important to adopt a long-term approach to health and fitness, recognizing that sustainable progress is built over time.

12. **Cultivating a positive mindset:** A mature perspective towards health and fitness involves cultivating a positive mindset. This means focusing on the progress that has been made, rather than fixating on any setbacks or obstacles. It also means practicing self-compassion and self-care, and recognizing that overall health and fitness is a journey rather than a destination.

By adopting these principles, you can develop a mature perspective towards health and fitness that supports your overall health and wellbeing throughout your life.

A mature perspective towards health and fitness involves creating healthy habits that are sustainable over time, recognizing the mind-body connection, prioritizing preventive measures, acknowledging individuality, and staying open to lifelong learning and flexibility.

Nothing Is Good in Excess – Achieve a great Balance in Everything

There is a great importance of moderation in all aspects of life, including workouts, fitness routines, diet, supplements, lifestyle, workstyle, and more. In order to maintain a healthy and balanced lifestyle, it is important to understand and implement this principle in every aspect of our lives. Let's explore each of these aspects in detail:

1. **Workouts and Fitness Routine:**

Exercise is important for our physical and mental well-being, but too much of it can lead to injury and burnout. It is important to have a balanced workout routine that includes a variety of exercises such as cardio, strength training, and flexibility training. For example, if you're doing strength training every day, make sure to give your muscles time to recover before working them again.

2. **Diet:**

Eating a balanced and healthy diet is essential for maintaining good health. However, overeating or consuming too much of a particular food group can lead to negative consequences. For example, eating too much sugar can lead to obesity and diabetes, while eating too much protein can put strain on your kidneys. It is important to consume a variety of foods in moderation, and to pay attention to portion sizes.

3. **Supplements:**

Supplements can be a useful addition to a healthy diet, but they should be taken in moderation. Taking too many supplements can lead to negative side effects and potentially harm your health. It is important to consult with a healthcare professional before taking any supplements, and to only take them as recommended.

4. **Lifestyle:**

Maintaining a healthy lifestyle involves more than just diet and exercise. It is important to also focus on other aspects of your life such as sleep, stress management, and social connections. For example, getting enough sleep is crucial for overall health and well-being, but sleeping too much can lead to negative consequences such as lethargy and a lack of productivity.

5. **Workstyle:**

Working hard is important for achieving success, but overworking can lead to burnout and negative health consequences. It is important to maintain a work-life balance by setting boundaries and taking breaks when needed. For example, taking breaks throughout the workday can help improve focus and productivity.

6. **Mental Health:**

Taking care of our mental health is just as important as taking care of our physical health. However, too much focus on our mental health can lead to an unhealthy preoccupation with negative thoughts and emotions. It is important to find a balance between acknowledging and addressing negative thoughts and emotions while also cultivating positive thoughts and emotions. For example, practicing gratitude and positive affirmations can help counteract negative thoughts and emotions.

7. **Social Life:**

Social connections are important for our overall well-being, but too much socializing can lead to exhaustion and burnout. It is important to find a balance between spending time with loved ones and taking time for yourself. For example, setting aside alone time to recharge can help prevent social burnout.

8. **Technology:**

Technology can be a helpful tool in many aspects of our lives, but too much screen time can lead to negative consequences such as eye strain and sleep disruption. It is important to find a balance between using technology for productivity and leisure while also taking breaks to give our eyes and brains a rest. For example, setting aside tech-free time before bed can help improve sleep quality.

9. **Hobbies:**

Hobbies are important for mental stimulation and personal growth, but too much focus on hobbies can lead to neglecting other important areas of life. It is important to find a balance between pursuing hobbies and taking care of responsibilities. For example, setting aside specific times for hobby activities can help ensure that other important areas of life are not neglected.

Balance is the key to maintaining a healthy and fulfilling lifestyle. By applying the principle of "nothing is good in excess – have balance in everything" to workouts, fitness routines, diet, supplements, lifestyle, and workstyle, you can achieve a more balanced and sustainable approach to health and wellness.

The principle of balance applies to every aspect of our lives, and finding the right balance can help us achieve a healthier, more fulfilling life.

Be Neutral towards every aspect of life:

The concept of neutrality suggests a state of non-attachment to any particular outcome or situation, allowing one to be free from the suffering that can come from identifying too closely with any given experience. This detachment can be seen as a way to cultivate a sense of inner peace and contentment, as it frees one from the constant fluctuations of pleasure and pain that arise from attachment and aversion.

From a philosophical perspective, this concept is closely tied to the principles of non-duality, which suggest that all phenomena are interconnected and ultimately arise from the same source. In this view, attachment and aversion arise from a false sense of separation between oneself and the world, and the ultimate goal of spiritual practice is to transcend this duality and recognize the fundamental unity of all existence.

Neutrality can also be seen as a way to cultivate equanimity, or a sense of balance and even-mindedness in the face of changing circumstances. By remaining neutral and non-reactive to external events, one is able to maintain a sense of inner stability and avoid being pulled off-centre by the ups and downs of life.

However, it is important to note that neutrality should not be confused with indifference or apathy. Rather, it is a way of being fully present and engaged with the world while maintaining a sense of inner detachment and non-judgment. This allows one to fully experience the richness and complexity of life without getting caught up in the drama and distractions that can lead to suffering.

Ultimately, the cultivation of neutrality requires a deep understanding of the nature of the mind and the nature of reality itself. It requires a willingness to let go of our preconceptions and beliefs and to embrace the mystery and uncertainty of existence with an open heart and mind. While it may not be easy to achieve this state of being, the rewards of inner peace, contentment, and freedom from suffering are well worth the effort.

THE END

www.ingramcontent.com/pod-product-compliance
Ingram Content Group UK Ltd.
Pitfield, Milton Keynes, MK11 3LW, UK
UKHW022209230426
12048UKWH00016BA/747